The Last Diet

By

Kelli Maw, MD, FAAFP, MPH

Edited by

Michael Premo

Recipes by

Thura (Peter) Han

Copyright © 2017 by Kelli Maw

Printed in the United States of America

ISBN-13: 978-1974229031

ISBN-10: 1974229033

First Printing, 2017

Acknowledgements

I would like to express my gratitude to Michael Premo for his invaluable editorial expertise, bibliographic research, and guidance in publishing this book. My deep appreciation goes to Thura (Peter) Han for his diligence in researching, creating, and selecting low-carb recipes. My gratitude goes to Dave Casey for the cover photograph, terrific support, extensive critique, and feedback. I thank Bernice Dalby greatly for the detailed review, advice, and encouragement. My heartfelt thanks to my mother, Dr. Khin Kyi, who said, "Just write the book." Last, but not least, I want to thank my patients, friends, and family for their support, especially those who gave me permission to write about their experiences and stories. All the names of those mentioned in this book have been changed.

Introduction

"The nine-inch stomach, the ocean within."

Translated from the Burmese saying,

"Thamodaya wun-ta-twa."

Why Bother Reading This Book?

This book is not about a 7 or 30-day plan to lose weight, nor will it make you a body builder or an Olympian. It is not a book of promises, like so many are offering out there. As of May 2017, a simple search on Amazon showed over 200,000 titles on weight loss. Many of them explain the best types of food to eat, provide some thoughtful recipes, and give many food options. We can also add to this growing list of books, other resources for weight loss such as the countless websites, the numerous gyms, the weight loss programs, and electronic gadgets available on the market. Yet, people are crossing over from normal to overweight and into obesity every day. Because of this, we live in paradoxical times—when our healthy choices and efforts don't seem to matter.

Fad diets come and go, and new gadgets pop up on the market every day. We learn new information about "super foods" and supplements frequently, and some are later found not to be what they seemed to be, or debunked. But some things that were true from the beginning of mankind are still true and will continue to be true for a very long time. A good amount of information in this book is based on these *lasting principles* which have become buried under the daily barrage of information. They will help you develop a state of awareness about how we interact with food, how the abundance of food has become detrimental to our health, and what we can do about it, which is why I named this book ***The Last Diet***.

The Burmese saying at the start of this chapter suggests that even though the stomach has limited physical capacity, its "needs" are endless. This is because our emotions and lifestyles drive our eating habits. We must eat to stay alive, but if we were simply eating to survive, then the problem of obesity and chronic disease would go away. But we are more sophisticated than that. We celebrate, and we mourn. We love, hate, laugh, praise, and cry. We must interact with people who we love as well as those we don't, but need to deal with, nonetheless. All these interactions may be associated with a meal, a feast or they simply give us a reason to eat. If we want to live life to the fullest, we must recognize this and look to the horizon for a long and healthy life.

Our cultural and personal habits have placed a third of Americans, children included, into dangerous territory. Every day, people are faced with choices about what to eat, what's good and bad for us, how much we should eat, and why it's important to pay attention to our weight. Yet, many people are unable to maintain healthy eating habits and more people are becoming obese than ever before. With this unprecedented epidemic comes a wide-range of chronic diseases and illness.

You're not alone, if you're like most people, who have tried to lose weight by following different diets and exercise plans, then gained it back. ***The Last Diet*** focuses on why diets don't work, and what to do about it. It also examines the psychological, social, and cultural reasons why people fail to lose weight even when they are successful in every other aspect of their life.

The weight loss industry has grown exponentially, along with our waist lines. While the industry offers additional tools and structure for losing weight, it has limitations. Diet and exercise are only part of the equation. Losing weight requires a thoughtful examination of our habits, our relationships, and the everyday stress that affects our ability to develop healthy eating habits.

This book is about understanding how to build a healthy lifestyle, so you can protect yourself from chronic disease and live longer. It is also about thoughtfully eating what you want, just not so much of it, so you can enjoy life and its celebrations. It's about your life as a journey and how to understand what you can do to manage your weight. As you will see, there is no magic diet or fat-burning super food. The potential and the power are in you, not the food, and this book is your companion for the journey ahead.

Who I Am

My interest in medicine and public health began in sixth grade, when I hung around my mother's operation suite and helped the staff clean and sterilize surgical instruments. My mother taught me how to tie surgical knots and understand the different suture material. After medical school and periods in various disciplines, I settled into a career in public health and family medicine and became attuned to the prevention of chronic diseases. Some memories from our childhood stand out, yet we never think about why they do for many years. For me, it felt like I was surrounded by widows: my grandmother, grand aunts, distant relatives, and family friends. Many of the men died young from heart attacks, leaving their wives, and sometimes young children, to fend for themselves. These men died in their peak years of productivity. They had *"bad hearts,"* which was taken for granted in my community. The widows would carry on as best as they could. Often, the children would step up and take care of their mothers before they were adults. Some of these families fell into poverty, some were taken in by relatives, or a relative would move in to help. Those that moved in with other families became the unpaid housekeepers and baby sitters, grateful to have a roof over their heads.

These were the humble women and families, some who eventually faded into oblivion as their hopes and dreams were ground to dust. Some lived their lives out in a state of "myet-nar–nge" or "small face," meaning in a humbled or lowered social standing. People called it destiny, and in my small corner of the world I knew women who silently held up more than half the sky. Granted, there were other instances such as divorce and accidents causing families to be torn apart, but it was the early cardiac deaths that left an impression on me. I wondered if the lives of the fractured families from my past would have been any different if they had been more knowledgeable about chronic disease prevention. I wondered if we, mere mortals, might have a certain level of control over our destinies.

My first opportunity to be involved in managing chronic diseases beyond the traditional clinical setting began when I was tasked with a project to address a chronic disease to reduce health disparities within the community. I chose diabetes because I felt that if my team and I could make a difference in the lives of with people living with diabetes, we could give them a fighting chance against all the complications that came with it, such as blindness, amputations, kidney failure, and heart disease. With a team of dedicated, certified nurse practitioners, nurses, nutritionists, and medical assistants, I saw first-hand, what people could achieve in the right setting with the right team support, and more importantly, with the right frame of mind.

A later opportunity arose for me to work one-on-one with obese and overweight patients who were trying to lose weight. When you interact with a population trying to achieve similar goals, you start noticing patterns. My team and I could usually identify which person would lose weight with little or no difficulty, and those who would need extra attention for different reasons. We were able to assess their knowledge and outlook during the first encounter.

For several years, I have been involved in conducting clinical research including clinical trials with weight loss medications. Some have the potential to control weight and control blood sugar at the same time. So, in the traditional clinical management setting, a team approach setting, and a clinical research setting, I have had the opportunity over the years, not just to study the effects of medications on disease, but the effects on people, and people's behavior—their psychological reactions—when on the medications. I have also had the privilege of getting to know some of their family dynamics, and to witness their anguish and their joy.

Why I Wrote This Book

From what I have written above, you will notice that I mention <u>frame of mind</u>, <u>family dynamics</u> and <u>emotions</u> as factors affecting our weight. Something else becomes evident as our society becomes more sophisticated, and that is, we live to a certain degree within the realm of a man-made reality. Most of the time, we love attractions such as theme parks, movies, and video games. But some of these environmental cues can subtly change the way we view ourselves and our environment. Sometimes, art imitates or dramatizes life. In the 1999 movie, *The Matrix*, a computer hacker discovers that people are living in a reality created by robots to control their minds[1]. Another example is *1984*, a book by George

Orwell, who wrote about how people's thinking and perceptions were manipulated and controlled. These are examples of how people can be easily influenced through marketing and propaganda. It makes us wonder why modern society has been fighting the battle against obesity, yet there have been no major victories for the general population.

There are so many diet books, diet plans, medical and surgical options, but we are still fighting an exhausting battle. Why the discrepancy? Who are the winners and losers? We will address this later, but for now, let's start by questioning our little piece of this world and our sphere of influence.

There is much is to be gained from having a questioning mind. In his book, *Power, Freedom and Grace*, Deepak Chopra describes a conversation with a patient. The patient gives him a strange look when he asks him why he wants to get better from his illness. Each time the patient answers, Chopra follows up with, "Why?" The patient wants to get better because he wants to get back to work, and if he can get back to work, he can make more money. Chopra leads him along the path one step at a time until the patient verbalizes something he has subconsciously wanted and worked towards without ever saying it. The ultimate answer is that the patient wants these things, because he wants to be happy. Chopra suggests that if happiness is the ultimate goal, why not just make it the primary goal. Embracing this concept, I want to add that there are many types of happiness, but the type of happiness that is accompanied by freedom and peace of mind is better than the short-lived happiness gained from immediate gratification.

If I were to ask someone why they want to lose weight, then ask additional questions like Dr. Chopra did, I am sure many will say that the final goal is happiness, freedom, and peace of mind. If we agree that evidence of such a state is a healthy and long life, then we should look at examples of people who have celebrated or are close to celebrating their 100th birthdays.

For generations, we have unsuccessfully tried to find the elusive fountain of youth. Meanwhile there are small pockets throughout the world where people have quietly become centenarians while leading simple lives. The island of Okinawa, Japan offers an excellent example. Also called the land of the immortals, the island boasts the largest number of centenarians in the world. They are of normal weight and look more than a decade younger than their ages. They stay active, lead productive lives and are known to eat only until they are ten-eighths full, a practice called *hara hachi bu,* or *hara hachi bun me.*

Another example of longevity is found among the Seventh Day Adventists in Loma Linda, California, many of whom have lived to see their 100th birthday. They abstain from smoking and alcohol and follow a vegan diet. Spirituality is thought to be a major factor for longevity in this group. People on the remote Mediterranean island of Ovodda, Sardinia, also enjoy long and healthy lives. Their longevity is thought to be the result of genetics.

The Okinawans' diet of seafood, protein and vegetables is different from the Mediterranean diet of people in Ovodda, which consists of proteins, cheese, olive oil, wine and vegetables. It is obvious that health and longevity is not determined by geography, culture, or a specific diet. If we look at the lifestyles of the centenarians, we see a common thread: disciplined eating, moderation, spirituality, staying active, and following a relatively simple lifestyle. In other words, there is a certain wisdom that brings happiness, freedom and a good life

At the most basic level, we eat to live. Food prolongs life. In other words, it is the *currency* we use to buy our time on this earth. A good way to think about this is to look at our retirement accounts. We believe that if we invest wisely, our 401Ks should provide for our financial needs and allow us to maintain a good standard of living for a long time. If food was treated like our 401Ks, and we learned how to use it wisely, perhaps we could achieve a long and high-quality life.

I realize that some people don't necessarily want to live to be over a hundred years old, and I am not sure that I would want to either. Regardless, we can agree that it is not the number of years we have left on this earth that matter, but the quality of those years. Whether I live to be a centenarian or not, I want to be as pain-free, active and take as few medications as possible. I want to enjoy this time with my family and not be a burden to them, and for them to be healthy as well. And this is also my wish for you.

Throughout this book, I will address matters related to our physical environment, our emotions, close relationships, facts about our body, and food. Longevity comes from a healthy lifestyle, not from simply following a diet, but, diets are an important part of the plan. In the next section, I review some of the popular diets that have been around for a while, so we can move beyond the questions and concerns about diets and focus on the issues that really matter.

The Named Diets

Working hard and sticking to a diet and then failing can be discouraging. Repeating this process multiple times make us wonder if any diet works at all, particularly when we have followed a difficult diet very closely, even though it didn't quite fit with our lifestyles. Because of this, we need to take an objective look at diets to see what research has found. There are large amounts of data available to help us understand which diets work and the ones that don't.

In 2013, an article in Consultant360[1] compared popular diets to answer the question whether these diets worked or not. The authors examined eight well known diets: Atkins (or low carbohydrate) diet, the Zone diet, Vegetarian, Vegan, Paleolithic, Gluten-free, Mediterranean, and the AARP New American Diet.

To begin, one of the most popular diets in the past couple of decades is the Atkins Diet[2], first developed by Dr. Atkins in 1958 and considered to be the original low-carb (carbohydrate) diet with no restrictions on fat intake and a higher protein intake than other diets. Dieters followed four phases, where all carbs are avoided in the beginning and gradually added back.

Along the lines of the Atkins diet is the Zone diet. It's a relatively low-carb diet, but further defines the proportions of the types of food to consume through percentage of daily intake: 40% carbohydrates, 30% proteins, and 30% fat. The reviewers noted that with both the Atkins diet and the Zone diet, people lost a significant amount of weight after a year, but the greatest amount of weight loss was seen in the first two months. An article[3] in the Journal of American Medicine (2014) discussed how both low carb and low-fat diets were associated with an approximate weight loss of 6 kg. (13.2 pounds) over a six-month period.

Vegetarian diets allow dairy and eggs, while vegan diets exclude animal products. Studies found that people on such diets had lower cholesterol and about half of the people were able to prevent diabetes. At one time, there was a concern about these diets not having enough nutrients such as certain vitamins and minerals, but nowadays, many foods are fortified with these nutrients. Another article[4] described how vegetarian diets reduced fat mass better than a diet where calories were simply restricted.

The idea behind the Paleolithic diet is that in the time of hunters and gatherers, humans ate mostly meats, fruits, vegetables and nuts, and the diet eliminates not just grains and legumes, but dairy products as well. While there are no long-term studies on this diet, the authors mentioned some health benefits and feeling full earlier.

The gluten free diet[4] is relatively new and has grown in popularity along with the increase in celiac disease awareness. Gluten is a mixture of proteins found in wheat, barley, oat, rye, and their hybrids. It provides the elastic texture when these products are cooked. Celiac disease is an autoimmune disorder, where people are allergic to gluten and the small intestine's ability to absorb nutrients is impaired, often causing malnutrition and weight loss. When gluten is removed from their diet, people with celiac disease gain weight.

On the other hand, in recent years, some people have associated their weight gain with gluten in their diet. Non-celiac gluten sensitivity[5,6] is a condition causing intestinal and non-intestinal symptoms from eating wheat but it is not currently clear whether this causes actual weight gain. Nevertheless, the food industry has responded by developing and labeling gluten free or gluten-friendly foods. Experts caution that such foods may not be necessarily better. For instance, gluten-free bread has a high glycemic index because it contains ingredients such as rice flour, tapioca, potato flour and cornstarch which makes our blood glucose rise very quickly.

The only way to decide whether gluten is the culprit is to avoid gluten for several months without changing anything else and to see if there is any weight-loss, then, adding it back to see if the weight returns. In clinical trials, this kind of process is called the "dechallenge" and "rechallenge" where a specific drug is established as a cause for a certain effect.

The Mediterranean diet mimics the diet of the Mediterranean region and allows fruits, vegetables, whole grains, legumes, fish, dairy, olive oil, and moderate amounts of meat and wine. Studies show that this diet benefits people living with diabetes and had benefits on weight.

The AARP New American Diet is a balanced approach to meals along with a healthy lifestyle. The emphasis is on reducing colon cancer and other types of cancer through whole grain consumption, which also maintains stable blood glucose levels. The premise of this diet is that food should be regarded as a preventative medicine.

What do professionals who help people with obesity and other chronic conditions eat? At a recent conference for health professionals specializing in obesity management, I heard two renowned cardiologists explain their personal dietary preferences. The first said that the Mediterranean diet worked best for him, while the other said that he had success on the low carb diet to control his blood pressure. In fact, when he came off the low-carb diet, his blood pressure started rising again, so he went back and had stayed on it ever since. He also noted that for some people who have successfully lost weight like him, there might be a level of "carbohydrate intolerance" where above a certain threshold, weight gain and other changes such as an increase in blood glucose levels and blood pressure may occur.

Among health care professionals who successfully managed their weight, many mention the low carb diet, followed by the Mediterranean diet and vegetarian diets. More importantly, whatever their preferred diet, they all stayed very active and exercised regularly. One thing most agree on, was that it was not so much the fats and oils, but the carbs in our diets that contributed to obesity.

Although they have their own unique characteristics, one thing in common among the named diets is the reduction of processed foods including processed meats, refined grains and sugar. In other words, they promote whole grains, or limit carbohydrates[8,9].

The Atkins diet, the Zone diet, the gluten-free diet, and the Paleolithic diet could be considered different varieties of low-carb diets. Even with the gluten-free diet, people may reduce consumption of carbohydrates to the point where the lowered carbohydrate intake would promote their weight loss. Of note, is that food products developed to specifically cater to certain diets can be more expensive than average products.

Because of the evidence that I have described, also from knowing what many experts recommend and eat themselves, and from my career experience, this book will emphasize a lower consumption of carbohydrates. But, one size doesn't fit all, and a good diet must meet individual needs. That being said, if there are so many diets around and scientific evidence that many of them do work and have many health benefits, then why is it so hard to lose weight? This is exactly what we will discuss in the next chapter.

1. Why Dieting Fails

"If you don't know where you're going, any road will take you there."
Cheshire cat, Alice in Wonderland

Browsing the news, we can see that a new diet fad pops up every six months or so. Many people will lose weight on these diets for a short period, yet fail to achieve their weight-loss goals. It is estimated that between 90 – 95% of dieters fail to achieve their goals and keep the weight off for longer than 5 years. On average, Americans start-and-stop these diets 4 times throughout a single year.

The reasons why fad diets fail range from the simple failure to count calories to the more complex issues related to lifestyle and changes in metabolism. One major reason why they fail is because our bodies crave the food we are accustomed to. When dieters introduce sudden changes to their eating and lifestyle, the body often responds with mood swings, head and body aches, and mental fatigue. These are not good feelings and cause many people to quit a diet within less than a week.

In countries under severe conditions such as famine or forced restrictions such as food rations, entire populations lose weight. In this country, when we go on a diet, we are essentially imposing artificial restrictions in an environment where food is abundant. This makes it very hard to stay focused on our goals, because wherever we turn, tasty food is available and plentiful. Dieting forces us to go against the natural flow of our environment and it ends up being an uphill battle. It makes us feel bad, so we tend to avoid them and make up reasons to not go on a diet, even though the reasons to lose weight are more important. Why do we do this?

Procrastination

You Want to lose Weight, but Never Get Around to It

Changing habits is hard even when our lives are calm and stable. It's harder when we are going through a major life event such as pregnancy, divorce or marriage. Our modern lifestyles demand that we make priorities. How can we change our eating habits when we are already navigating other changes? For instance, we step on the scale in the morning and realize that we have gained another couple of pounds. Before we can shake that feeling of frustration, it's time to get going, so we grab our stuff and head out the door. As we drive to work, we brace ourselves and prepare for the unfinished business waiting there. We decide to be prepared for a busy day, so we stop at a fast food restaurant. Several items look good, and we know they're not all necessarily healthy, but it helps us through the morning, so we pick up a few things. A couple of minutes later, we are on our way. For many of us, this has become our routine. And we like that there is no need to worry about making breakfast, because we can walk right into work and get started.

Routines can be a good thing. They give us some control over our hectic lives. But how that routine is designed may make or break your weight management efforts. Changing a well-functioning routine is hard, especially when those changes affect others around you and you know they are going to resist the changes. Just the thought of going through the emotional effort makes us want to avoid it. So, we put off losing weight. We say, "I'll start eating better tomorrow".

We also make excuses about the time it takes to count calories and keep track of what to eat. The time and effort it takes to go on a diet is put off to the next day, and the next. Eventually, a week has gone by and the diet is forgotten. A month goes by and the thoughts of losing weight are long gone, and losing weight is no longer a priority.

Diet Fatigue

You Begin a Diet, Do Well in the Beginning,
but Fail when Fatigue Sets in

We all know that food is fuel for the body. Our bodies rely on the vital nutrients in food to sustain our daily activities. When the number of calories is significantly reduced, the body has less fuel to turn into energy and we feel fatigued. Because there are a lot of expectations at work or home, some people can't have this feeling of sluggishness throughout their day. Fewer calories also affect our ability to focus or stay on task. This is why people on very low-calorie diets (VLCD) and eat less than 700 calories per day should do so only on a temporary basis and have proper guidance and support.

Obesogenic Environments

Where You Live and Work is not Conducive to Losing Weight

I have helped several people who worked in the food industry, whose jobs required them to be surrounded by food all day. Some were involved in developing and testing delicious, new recipes. Others owned their own restaurant or bakery. Tasting was an important part of their job.

Plus, the hours were long and stressful. They would go on a diet and lose some weight, only to gain it back. All of them were eager to lose weight and made tremendous attempts, but very few achieved significant and sustained weight loss unless they had structured support. None of them were in a situation where they could quit their jobs.

Obesogenic environment[1] is a relatively new term emerging from research and a better understanding of the growing obesity epidemic over the past decade. It describes the physical and cultural surroundings that promote gaining weight at work, in the community or at home. People in the food industry are surrounded by food all day and are constantly bombarded by food messaging. Their struggles to lose weight are constant battles against their lifestyle choices and from being immersed in obesogenic environments. Even if we don't work in the food industry, we are subjected to this environment too. Pay attention when you are driving, and you will see that fast food restaurants are strategically placed near intersections, signaling quick and easy access to food. This contributes to impulsive purchases of high-calorie, high-fat foods.

Portion Distortion Disorder

Your Eyes Are Bigger than Your Stomach

In the past 20 years, portion sizes at restaurants have gotten larger. A great example of this is soda (pop). Prior to the 1950s, Coca-Cola was sold in bottles with one size—6.5 ounces. Today, plastic 20-ounce bottles are the norm, almost tripling the number of calories. Fast food is presented as a good deal when it includes the fries and soda to make it a meal, yet the a la carte sandwich holds enough calories for one meal. Restaurants have to fill their plates with food to show value. There can be enough food on that one plate to feed two, sometimes three people. Portion distortion can be directly tied to our expectations for quality and value. What is a good deal for our wallets may be a bad deal for our waistlines.

This is one of the reasons behind not being able to lose weight. I remember reading how Parisian women managed to stay slender while eating croissants, baguettes, and drinking wine. Yet, bread and wine are a major "no-no" in many diets. I also remember a story about an American who was invited to dinner with a French family. After some good conversation, his stomach was rumbling, and he was more than ready for the meal especially when he heard they had prepared a five-course meal. They finally sat down to eat, and the dish in front of him had two small carrots. His face visibly fell, because he couldn't hide his disappointment. It hadn't occurred to him until then that people stayed slender by eating small portions. These are examples of what we've come to expect when we sit down to eat, pointing out our cultural differences with food.

Calories: Under – Over

Underestimate Calories Eaten, Overestimate Calories Burned

In the United States and other developed countries, we are blessed with an abundance of food. This overabundance has led to generous portions, more food on the table and calories eaten. Many would agree that counting calories is next to impossible, because the nutritional listings on packages are too confusing, and nutritional data is not always available. Because of this, people often underestimate the number of calories eaten.

Besides, different foods are digested, absorbed and metabolized differently.

Now, we add physical activity and exercise into the equation which greatly influences the number of calories burned. We rarely consider all the factors required in calculating our energy use.

Karen and Conner, who eat out about three times a week, are a good example. They typically share an appetizer, order some drinks, have their own entrees, then end the meal with dessert. On the weekend, they work in their yard for a couple hours, cutting the hedge and pulling weeds. Because they "had a good workout," they feel justified in going to an all-you-can-eat Chinese buffet. Periodically, they express their frustration at their continued weight gain despite being active. Counting calories in both directions is difficult.

Gadgets

Relying on Technology or External Aids

Fitness trackers and smartphone apps have become popular tools in the pursuit to lose weight and become healthier. Many apps provide quick answers to questions about nutrition and help account for daily caloric intake. Fitness trackers do the hard math in calculating the calories burned while exercising. The price range for these varies from several dollars to hundreds of dollars. They can help people lose weight when used correctly, but a recent study[2] shows they are less effective than hoped to be. People wearing fitness trackers lost less weight than those who monitored their own activity. Researchers found that people relied on the technology and developed a false sense of security, but when people relied on themselves they were more diligent in keeping track of their progress. I have met more people who have been successful with nothing more than a simple scale, a servings size guide and a food diary than some who wear the latest gadgets.

This reminds me of a good friend who has struggled with her weight. At one time, she had sought my advice and lost some weight, but gave up in the long run and gradually regained the weight she lost. One day, we met at a neighborhood restaurant for brunch. She kept looking at her watch, so I asked her what she was checking for. She said, "It's my fitness gadget buzzing me." I had to ask, "Buzzing you for what?" She said it was synchronizing with her phone and set off the alarm for how many steps she had taken. She wasn't on a diet, so I asked, "Why did you get it?" To my surprise, she said she didn't, but a couple of friends gave it to her, so that they could synchronize their activities to challenge each other to exercise more. I asked her if it was working and she said, "No." She said it cost about $160. I told her I could think of a lot of other things to spend $160 on, like a dozen brunches. We laughed and ate our meals. At least a gadget worn on the wrist takes up less room than a piece of gym equipment that is not used and takes up half of your study, garage or basement. Gadgets will be as effective as you allow them to be—no more and no less.

We Forget What We Ate

Yesterday's Calories Are Still There, Even If You've Forgotten Them

There is such a thing as the Yesterday, Today, and Tomorrow bush. It grows along the edges of my yard. Once a year, it blooms in early summer with little purple flowers. After a few days, the flowers fade a bit to lavender, then after a few more they turn completely white before dying. I think about these bushes whenever I talk about counting calories. In a way, our habits and obligations during the holidays resemble this pretty shrub.

The day before Thanksgiving, we have a potluck luncheon at the office. Everyone brings a dish or dessert. The following day we eat with our families, usually a large turkey with all the trimmings. There is enough food to last a full week—the leftovers seem endless. After Thanksgiving is Black Friday, the annual kick off for holiday shopping season. It's easier to grab a bite to eat while running around town picking up last minute gifts. The festivities continue throughout December, gathering after gathering with coworkers and friends, always centered around a meal and drinks. Before we know it, we're celebrating Christmas, then eating Christmas leftovers. And, we can't forget New Year's Eve and New Year's Day celebrations.

As each day brings us closer with family and friends, securing our bonds that bring us great joy and happiness, we realize it's time to make our resolutions. For many of us the resolutions will be just like the year before—to lose 10 pounds or more. When we try to lose weight, we tend to forget about what we ate the day before, but those calories don't forget. The food we ate during the holiday season tends to hang on, just like those little purple flowers hanging on for a little while longer, only changing their color. It is those forgotten calories that form little folds and love handles around the waist and elsewhere. I use the holidays as an example because the effect on our waistlines is rather obvious, but for some of us, similar scenarios can happen at any time of the year, or even throughout the year.

Lifestyle

Choosing a Diet That Is Incompatible with Everyday Life

The National Institute of Health and Centers for Disease Control[3] suggests making some lifestyle changes that affect diet and increase exercise. The recommendations focus on alternative choices to foods high in sodium, sugar and fat. These are relatively minor and require some thought and planning. According to these suggestions, combined with regular exercise, people could potentially maintain or lose weight. Unfortunately, many people feel that they need to make dramatic measures to quickly counteract months or even years of poor eating habits.

Here are a couple examples of these dramatic changes to drive this point home. One American family was inspired by Okinawans and what they ate. The family went on a diet of fish, tofu, seaweed and vegetables. After a month or so, they gave up. Japanese culture, especially on the Island of Okinawa in the Pacific, is very different from American culture. The changes to their lifestyle through this diet were too dramatic. I wondered, rather than making such a drastic change, if they had simply adopted the philosophy of the Okinawans and ate their usual food with small modifications, until they were eight-tenths full, perhaps they could have a sustainable dietary plan. But then, we would have to know what eight-tenths is like.

Some people take drastic measures for a medical reason, like supporting needs of their child or spouse. There was a TV show about a family who gave up sugar due to a medical condition in one of the family members. At the end of the show, one of the kids commented on how much he missed ice cream. Dieting is difficult enough, but changing entire ways of living is nearly impossible, because we often crave what we can't have.

Too Boring

The Routine Is Monotonous and Lacks Variety

The Atkins diet was tremendously popular for a while. People on this diet were allowed to eat as much protein and high fat foods as they wanted without counting portions or calories. This had a universal appeal to it. Plus, American diets were also high in protein and fat when compared to other developed nations, so it was a natural fit to our culture. I saw many people lose weight on this diet, but once they stopped, all their weight came back. I have not yet met anyone who said goodbye to all carbohydrates—forever. Dieting suggests routine and monotony through restricting choices. We crave choices and options. The entire economy is built upon this premise and taking away choices is seen as a bad thing.

Costs Outweigh the Benefits

The Money and Time Spent Requires Too Much Effort

Sometimes it is out of necessity that people cannot stay on a diet. If you have a large family and are on a limited budget, you will naturally have to mix cheaper ingredients into the meals. Low-cost items that make us feel full after eating are typically carbohydrates, such as bread, pasta, rice and potatoes. As previously mentioned, there are so many diets to choose from, but our success depends on how well we stick with them and whether they fit our lifestyle, budget and the needs of our families.

Commercial diet programs, often advertised by a celebrity spokesperson, can be expensive. They may help in the short term, but it may be difficult to stay on the programs in the long term. Sometimes, the cost is not monetary. Personalized weight-loss programs provide close monitoring and require frequent visits. Even though people may benefit from the monitoring, it may be difficult to make the time commitment.

Take a moment and think of the words we associate with losing weight. A diet is a noun—a thing—simply a set of guidelines regarding food and weight loss. To say, "a diet fails" is the wrong assumption to make. Is it the diet—a thing—that fails or the process that creates challenges for us? Diet is also a verb, and many of us see it as a struggle, something we do to go against the grain of our everyday lives to achieve a weight loss goal. The more the diet differs from the way we live our real lives, the more difficult it is to sustain.

If you are a wonderful baker and you have always baked the best brownies for your grandchildren, it's hard to say no when they clamor for treats. We also treat ourselves with food, because we worked hard and earned the right to reward ourselves. Denying ourselves life's simple pleasures feels wrong. Then one day, our health provider tells us we are pre-diabetic and must be careful about what we eat. Along with other chronic diseases related to being overweight and obese, this is becoming a more common occurrence for baby boomers, adults and even some children. Our failure to lose weight can have a lasting effect on our bodies and make us more prone to diseases that go beyond simple aches and pains. Obesity makes us more susceptible to disease for many reasons and we will review them in the following chapter.

2. The Connection Between Obesity and Disease

"Laugh, and the whole world laughs with you. Weep, and you
weep alone.
For this sad old earth, must borrow its mirth, but has enough
sorrow of its own."

"Solitude" by Ella Wheeler Wilcox

From the public service announcements on the radio to the
billboards that line the highways, nearly everyone has seen or heard about
weight loss, weight control, and getting in shape. The reason, simply put,
is that we have an epidemic in this country. Gaining weight often goes
along with social activities. There is lots of goodwill and camaraderie. It
is associated with pleasant feelings and it is painless – to a point. In
contrast, losing weight is a lonely and uncomfortable journey. Two-thirds
of US adults are overweight, and one-third are obese or have a body mass
index (BMI) of 30 or more. Extreme obesity affects 1 in 20 adults.
Substantial weight gain has become a problem and more people are
becoming aware of it through public service campaigns.

Some of the announcements are advertisements for weight loss
clinics and plastic surgery. Additionally, trendy boot camps and gyms
provide a place to lose weight. They offer services to lose weight, to
reduce the effects of aging, and slow or prevent the progression of many
types of diseases.

Obesity was officially recognized as a disease in 2013[1]. There was
some controversy regarding this at the time, but here is one way to look at
it. Disease comes from the combination of two words, "dis" and "ease,"

meaning, not being at ease, or having discomfort. People who are overweight or obese sometimes tell me how physically uncomfortable they feel even though they may not have a chronic disease condition. They feel very different from the time when they did not have to carry the extra weight.

The problems associated with excessive weight gain are not just physical. Mental and social health and well-being are affected as well. It is not unusual for someone to suffer emotionally from the negative perceptions of weight, and the vicious cycle of emotional eating. Diseases associated with obesity affect the circulatory, musculoskeletal system and digestive system, and some cancers have been associated with excess weight gain. One of the most common diseases is type 2 diabetes. Other conditions include osteoarthritis, cardiovascular disease, and high cholesterol.

Chronic Diseases Associated with Obesity

Unfortunately, some people will come to acknowledge the effects of excessive weight gain after they are diagnosed with a physical disease. Failure to lose weight over the years may result in any of the following diseases:

Heart Disease	Kidney Disease
Type 2 Diabetes	Pancreatitis
Stroke	Fatty Liver Disease
Obstructive Sleep Apnea	Neuropathy
Cancer	High Blood Pressure
Gallstones	Heart Attack
Osteoarthritis	

Many of these diseases are painful. For instance, gall stones cause painful blockage in the bile duct. Neuropathy from diabetes typically starts as tingling, numbness and pain in the toes in the early stages spreads further up the foot and leg as the disease progresses in a "glove and stocking" pattern. Each of these has a level of pain associated with them. The pain is a clear signal for change. It's the body's way of saying, "Stop! It's time to see a doctor." I'd like to expand this discussion a little more by talking in depth about a few specific diseases.

Type 2 Diabetes

The rise in type 2 diabetes coincides with the rise in obesity. It's the seventh leading cause of death in the United States. A person's family history may have a role in developing type 2 diabetes, but low activity and poor diet are the common causes.

All carbohydrates from our diet must be broken down into the simplest form of carbohydrate, glucose, before it can be used by our bodies. The absorption begins in the intestines, after which glucose enters the bloodstream. It still has to get into our body's cells where it will be converted into energy. As part of this process, the pancreas produces insulin which transports glucose into our body's cells where it is converted into a form that is usable for energy or stored in the liver and fat cells.

In type 2 diabetes, the body's insulin supply cannot keep up with the abnormally high levels of sugar in the blood. This means that every organ and blood vessel in the body is bathed in sugar. Over time, this causes damage to the small blood vessels and nerve endings. At later stages of the disease, major vital organs that depend on these blood vessels and nerves become damaged. When the blood supply to the heart is damaged, heart attacks occur. Damage to the retinal vessels of the eyes can lead to blindness, and when the nerves and blood vessels of the feet become destroyed, it can lead to amputations. These are all painful and or devastating conditions.

But it is not all bad news. According to a Guidelines article in the American Family Physician[2], people at high risk for developing type 2 diabetes can significantly reduce the rate of diabetes onset with intensive lifestyle modification programs. To achieve these results, changes to diet and exercise need to happen as soon as the risk is recognized, along with frequent monitoring by a health care professional[3]. Three large-scale randomized placebo-controlled studies were conducted in China, Finland, and the United States to see if intensive lifestyle changes could help prevent diabetes in people who had prediabetes. The results showed that almost half of the people in the studies were able to prevent the development of diabetes. Regardless of culture, nationality and diet, these studies show how positive changes to lifestyle habits can lower weight and prevent a potentially life-threatening disease.

Metabolic Syndrome and Cardiovascular Disease

The leading cause of death in the United States, and a major concern throughout the world, cardiovascular disease has many causes. One particular form of cardiovascular disease results from metabolic syndrome, sometimes called syndrome X^4, which is caused by obesity. People with large amounts of abdominal fat have larger waists. The fat in the abdomen becomes resistant to insulin, blood sugar level increases, and diabetes can develop. Large amounts of fat also mean higher levels of bad cholesterol, and lower levels of good cholesterol. All of this in combination leads to deposits of fat lining and narrowing our blood vessels (atherosclerosis), high blood pressure and ultimately, heart attacks and strokes. Nobody would argue that these are not painful conditions, and the consequences can drastically change our lives and that of our families.

Osteoarthritis (Degenerative Joint Disease)

Depending on our activities and wear and tear on our joints, we are susceptible to osteoarthritis as we age, but people carrying excess weight suffer more pain from it. With age, the cartilage in our joints becomes more brittle and less resilient. Excessive wear and tear can cause damage, inflammation and loss of cartilage until the joint becomes *"bone-on-bone."* This degenerative change can happen in any of our joints, sometimes not even sparing the joints of the neck. As one expert put it, exaggerating somewhat, if you have been an agreeable person all your life and nodded your head a lot, you might even get arthritic neck pain as you age. The neck is a weight bearing structure since it supports our head, but the weight it carries is nowhere near what our knees and hips endure through our lifespans.

We take our knees for granted until the pain starts. When you think about it, these two small structures, with a surface area barely larger than the size of our palms support our entire body from the knee up. According to the arthritis organization[5], each pound of body weight gain turns into four pounds of pressure on the knees. A gain in 10 pounds of body weight turns into 40 pounds of pressure on the knees whenever we are standing or walking, and worse, when we climb stairs. For example, if we sat with a 5-pound bag of potatoes on our lap the moment we start walking while carrying the bag—the pressure on the knee is the equivalent of 20 pounds —because of the way pressure is distributed. You can see how taking a few pounds off your body weight can take the pressure of your knees, hips and back in a very significant way. People who were able to do this have often told me how it was a pleasure not to feel pain with every footstep.

Cancer

Cancer has always had ominous implications, and we associate it with pain, suffering and in many cases, death. Some cancers such as breast and colon cancer can be associated with genetics. New research[6] shows that colorectal cancers are now thought to be related to microbes in the gastrointestinal tract. Regardless of the cause, a diagnosis of cancer leaves us with a sense of despair and helplessness. In many cases, we feel that death is inevitable. On the other hand, if we could have done something to reduce, modify or eliminate our risk, I am sure many of us would. For instance, some people who have the breast cancer gene choose to have mastectomies to prevent cancer, and people who have precancerous polyps in the colon have them removed before the polyps turn into cancer. In other words, we can modify our level of risk for certain cancers. One of the benefits from managing our weight and avoiding obesity in the long term is that it can reduce our risk of cancers known to be associated with obesity such as breast cancer, endometrial cancer, prostate cancer, and colorectal cancer.

Pain Points

We think we bear the pain of physical and emotional illness alone, yet our family and loved ones inevitably share in the consequences of our disease. Some conditions associated with obesity are painless, until they're not. These include high blood pressure, high cholesterol, type 2 diabetes, heart disease and some cancers as mentioned above. They are all silent killers that can sneak up and strike us despite the best available medicines.

We naturally pay attention when something hurts, and not so much when it doesn't, therefore we suffer the long-term consequences that come with some unpleasant things.

Type 2 diabetes is so insidious that it can start years before it becomes evident. If it is not controlled, complications may manifest as actual pain in the legs, or loss of vision. As the disease progresses, some people may no longer be able to work, losing their independence and becoming a burden to their families. Conditions like obesity and associated diseases such as diabetes, heart disease and high blood pressure are, to a certain degree, perpetuated by us and therefore in some instances can be prevented or controlled.

Several years ago, I had a discussion with an airline pilot. A rule by the Federal Aviation Administration for sleep apnea was going to disqualify him for from flying a plane. Specifically, having a BMI of 40 or more can dramatically raise the occurrence of sleep apnea. He had to lose weight fast or else be grounded. This is an example of a pain point. He was forced to change his lifestyle to continue being a pilot. Quitting his job was not an option because his family depended on his ability to fly. Sometimes, the pain from weight gain is both physical and economical.

While more research is being done on the effects of excessive weight, the list of diseases continues to grow. The conditions discussed in this chapter are more common and should be of concern for anyone with a body mass index (BMI) of 30 or more. Another reason to take charge of our health is for the sake of family and friends. A younger person struck down by the consequences of obesity may have to be buried by their elderly parents, leaving the elderly to fend for themselves. Or they may live a long but sickly life, becoming a burden to their own families. Although the pain in obesity may not be obvious early on, the pains caused by obesity have a way of hurting not just us physically, but those who love us, as well.

3. Getting Motivated – Staying Motivated

"Mind over Matter. If you don't mind, it doesn't matter."

Mark Twain

"In order to change, we must be sick and tired of being sick and

tired."

Author Unknown

In the previous chapter, I discussed several painful conditions associated with obesity and chronic disease. Now, I will discuss how to get motivated to lose weight. I admit that when I hear the word "motivation," the image that comes to mind is that of someone scampering away before someone else gives them a swift kick in the behind. But sometimes that is exactly what we need to get started.

The decision to lose weight is an important one. Yet, it is easier said than done, because it can be a long and difficult process, and many of us struggle to find the spark to get started and to maintain the desire and ambition to lose weight and stay motivated. Many people fail to begin a weight-loss plan, either procrastinating and putting it off for another day, or they fail to follow through on their plan because they did not have the motivation to achieve their goals. Research has shown how diet plans are equally effective and have the same chance of success, because no single plan is more successful than the others. After analyzing numerous studies, researchers concluded that motivation was the key to this phenomenon and successful completion of a diet plan was determined upon whether a person was motivated to achieve their goals or not. This leads to a very important question for anyone who wants to lose weight: Why do you want to lose weight? What's in it for you?

For many, I know this is a difficult question. It goes beyond simply setting a goal. It's a plan for the "future me" and continues well beyond the achievement of those goals. I began the book with many reasons why people fail to lose weight, including the difficulty in getting motivated even when we know the importance of maintaining a healthy weight.

The Damage from Having a Victim Mentality

Modern life is such that we must filter out certain things in our busy daily lives to make it through each day. Seemingly unimportant and harmless things build up over time until things get out of control. Sometimes, this loss of control feels like a hurricane went through your house and left you surrounded by damage and destruction. Whether it is a slow erosion or a sudden catastrophe, the results can nonetheless be devastating. In some instances, things are truly beyond our control and at other times, it is because we did not make corrections earlier.

As mentioned earlier, carrying additional weight is associated with several painful chronic medical conditions. A quick and easy solution would be to treat these conditions as they arise with medications or surgery, but we must decide how long we want to take these medications, and whether that is a good long-term solution. I know people whose medication list goes on for five pages, and I think it must take a lot of effort to take so many medications. Some bitterly complain about the side effects of the medications and the need to take even more medications to treat these side effects.

A person has the choice to not do anything, and let life take its course. What would happen if we decided not to change a thing? If we do, then the list of medications, the ailments and the intensity of pain would simply continue to build. Making no decision is a decision. Our actions and inactions come with consequences. There is no way around it.

Diets are about making changes and many people are fearful of change. Why? Because, routine is comfortable and reliable, and going through changes shakes up those feelings of comfort and stability. Fred Kofman's explanation of victim mentality[1], where some people think they are powerless and at the mercy of external circumstances, speaks to the reason for lack of motivation in many areas of our lives including losing weight.

He explains how victim mentality allows people to feel good about themselves when things go wrong by blaming others and avoiding responsibility through maintaining innocence. He also points out that by claiming innocence, people are admitting they feel powerless, and I would add, that they would prefer to remain naïve.

During a lunch with a colleague and her family, her husband, a paramedic, spoke about the people he sometimes saw when they called the ambulance. Some would say to him afterward, "I went to the emergency room (ER) and they didn't do anything for me." It always amazed him, because when he asked specific questions, they would say the staff at the ER did lab tests, x-rays, and other imaging studies and gave them medications before discharging them or admitting them. Yet, when he pointed out that they did receive all the correct treatment, they would still grimace and say, "Well, not really." They wanted to remain a victim of their circumstances. This is the mentality that Kofman describes as an easy way to feel sorry for oneself and blame others, because *bad things do happen and the events and circumstances are real.*

Kofman points out that when people avoid responsibility, they also avoid the ability to respond appropriately to get themselves out of the situation. I see such people, who typically tell the person in front of them that whoever the last person that tried to help "didn't do anything for me." This mental outlook is also applied to inanimate objects as well, like diet plans and medications. It's often said that attitude is like a flat tire—unless it's changed, that person is going nowhere.

The Discomfort of Salvaging Your Life

People are temporarily in a state of shock and grief when a tornado, hurricane or earthquake devastates their homes or towns. They walk around what used to be their homes that had suddenly been taken away from them. They feel a sense of loss, grief, anger and disbelief as they pick through shattered memories. They try to get their bearings back and see if anything is salvageable. As people pick through the rubble of their homes trying to piece things together to start over, they walk through the history of their lives. When people realize that they have to change their eating habits because their weight has become out of control, they reflect on the events that led them to this point. There is a sense of being vulnerable, like someone who suddenly loses their home and sanctuary.

If your entire family has adopted a lifestyle that promotes obesity, and you suddenly decide to lose weight, you might feel like an outcast, and they might not feel comfortable with what you are doing. It's hard to break out of the status quo and there may be some feelings of guilt and lack of confidence associated with it.

Rosie's experience is a good example. She was approximately 70 pounds over her healthy weight. She once told me, "I let things go for a very long time because I had too much going on in my life. Each time I gained weight, I would go shopping for larger size clothes. I was happy for a little bit each time I found something I liked and looked flattering and fashionable, but then I outgrew it after a short while and I would have to go shopping again for yet a larger size. In the meantime, I was also developing back and knee pain, chest pain, high blood pressure and never really felt good. One day, I looked at the mirror and asked myself *why do I have to keep spending more and more money on clothes and medication just to hate myself?"*

These were powerful words and served as her first step to making changes in her life. The pounds had crept up slowly, but the realization that the damage had been done and she was in a bad situation hit her suddenly when the expenses had spun out of control. She was in debt, in pain, and extremely frustrated. The medical and imaging bills had piled up. She looked at her closets and they were spilling over with clothes that were too tight for her after she had worn them a couple of times.   Then there were the pictures of happier days when she could run and play with her children and go on long hikes with her husband. She felt a sense of loss of how life used to be, and how the quality of her life had been taken away from her.

Getting Our Bearings: Anchoring Ourselves through Motivation

Let's look at the different types of motivation[2]. Using rewards or punishment to lose weight is called **external motivation**. I have met people whose employers introduced work place wellness programs with rewards and subtle punishments. With one model, the people were placed in groups and the groups competed to see which one lost the most weight, with a cash reward going to the winning group. The external motivations were the employer's authority to implement the program, form the groups, and the cash incentive. Obviously, the moment the cash incentive went away, the game was over. External motivation is fleeting and doesn't work in the long term. Simply put, when someone has the authority to give you motivation, they also have the power to take it away.

Now, let's look at how non-external motivations work. For some people in this group, the idea of being pressured to lose weight went against their grain. Some felt like this was an imposition, and they felt guilty if they lost less weight than expected for the week. This kind of motivation is called **introjected motivation**, and they couldn't wait for the wellness program to be over. It wasn't that they didn't want to lose weight, they just didn't want to do it and still feel guilty and stressed every week. They felt that if they didn't go along with the plan, they would be resented by the rest of the group as not being team players.

On the other hand, there were some who simply thrived on the group interactions. They loved that the employer provided nutritional counseling sessions and free gym memberships. They valued the learning process and enjoyed seeing their blood test results improve each time they went for checkups. They were driven by **internal motivation.** Internal motivation and introjected motivation are related in that they both come from within us, but one is characterized by negative feelings and dread, while the other is characterized by positive feelings.

The last form of motivation is called **identified motivation**, when someone has identified a need to change, and truly wants to change but has not yet taken action because of their circumstances. A good example of this is a woman named Melissa, who leads a busy modern lifestyle with her husband and kids. Over the years, she noticed that they had gained weight. Her husband started experiencing foot pain when going up and down the stairs in their 3-story house. He considered testosterone replacement treatment, because some of his friends had suggested that it might be the reason he was not losing weight. He also thought that it might be his thyroid. Although Mellissa didn't have a problem with him checking his testosterone and thyroid tests, she felt she knew one big reason behind his weight and physical problems. His work included a lot of business lunches and dinners, where food was abundant, and everyone was expected to eat and have a few drinks while making business deals. There is irony in his situation, because when he was younger, he was a body builder and was very knowledgeable about nutrition and weight loss. Melissa and her family were victims of their own success.

Leading such busy lives, she could see the many opportunities for exercise that had been contracted out, such as yard work, most laundry needs and the housekeeping. She knew she had to do something about her own weight, so she and her daughter contemplated signing up with a mail-order diet meal plan.

The family typically went out to eat on the weekends and he would be upset at them for eating out so much and blaming it as the reason they couldn't lose the weight. Mellissa said they went out as a family just once each weekend, while he ate at restaurants several times a week for business. Mellissa knew that the meal plan was only a short-term solution. She wasn't even sure how she was going to handle the weekend restaurant meals while trying to stay on the plan. And his lack of encouragement made her think hard about what was life was going to be like afterwards and how she would stay motivated. She had what we discussed as identified motivation, while he was in the victim mentality mode.

We will revisit these kinds of challenges in later chapters, such as *Zones of Influence* and *Modern Family Dynamics*. This section is about how you can gather your thoughts and identify what truly motivates you. When weight loss is connected to something you value, it has meaningful purpose. The emotional connection and being able to focus on the task at hand drives us to achieve the goals we set for ourselves. More and more research[3] is backing this theory to the point of it being a crucial indicator of whether we will begin a weight loss program and stick with it or fail.

The Advantage of Having a Mindset for Success

Advantage is a word used to describe "a condition giving a greater chance of success." An example from sports might be a tall person who decides to play professional basketball or volleyball or a bilingual person who speaks a native language who becomes an interpreter. We all agree that changing habits is not easy, but necessary. Those who understand what motivates them have an advantage over those who don't by having a source of strength to draw from and can position themselves for greater success. According to Albert E. Gray[4], "The one factor that seems to transcend all the rest is the ability to focus on getting the important things done regardless of the enjoyment factor within the assignment. Successful people don't necessarily like doing them either. But their disliking is subordinated to the strength of their purpose."

Those who can prioritize and stick to their priorities have a clear advantage. Some may associate making priorities and having discipline as a very rigid lifestyle. Mark Twain said, *"The only way to keep your health is to eat what you don't want, drink what you don't like, and do what you'd rather not."* Twain's quote is a great example of how many of us feel when choosing healthier lifestyles and eating habits. He may not have thought very highly of having a healthy lifestyle, but he lived to be 75 years-old during a time when the average life expectancy was 50.

The way we think about diets borders on grieving about the loss of good things in our lives, such as the taste of good food and cocktails, but managing your weight doesn't have to be a life committed to eating only things you don't like.

What do we have in us that can be a great advantage? One of the things I admire the most about Americans is our fierce, independent spirit. There are many stories of people who started from extreme poverty and became very successful. They started from having nothing, sometimes not even shoes, and worked their way to wealth through sheer determination and the desire to be independent. I have seen this spark remain long after they have lost many other things. Some of my patients with memory loss have forgotten their home address and sometimes, what day of the week it is. Some have trouble recognizing family members and get lost in their neighborhood grocery stores that they have been going to for years. Yet, there is something that they often ask me. They ask when they will get their driver's license or their pilot's license back. Independence is such a deeply rooted trait that even when other things have disappeared, the yearning for independence remains. We don't like being at someone's mercy. It is something we take for granted, but I like to think that it is this desire that has contributed to the term, "The American Dream." You may have forgotten about it, but it's still in you. If you have made the connection between health and independence and remember the times when you rose above difficult situations, then you can revive this capability.

What if we weren't born with a physical or mental advantage or mindset for success? I would argue that one of the most important factors for success, regardless of our innate abilities, is the intentional development of discipline. For some, discipline is almost second nature, but for the rest of us, it doesn't come easy. This is where we need reminders and tools to help us. Discipline does not necessarily mean rigid rules. But it does mean understanding limits, to avoid making excuses for oneself, taking responsibility, and in the words of Augusta F. Kantra, "discipline is choosing between what you want now and what you want most". The right knowledge goes a long way towards developing discipline. Learning about your body mass index (BMI), counting calories, and understanding how food work are all tools to help you maintain discipline. Tools such as planning meals, understanding your healthy body weight and how calories work are needed for a disciplined approach to managing your weight. This is no different than learning the rules and knowing where the goal posts are in sports. These in turn greatly enhance your motivation.

Planning and managing your meals around your work day as well as around holidays and vacations is a form of discipline. So is deciding to lose the five pounds of holiday weight before it becomes fifteen. Hiring a personal trainer or nutritionist, joining a gym or a weight loss program, are all methods and tools to help us have a certain level of discipline. But how do you keep it going in the long term?

Using Leverage to Go Even Further

Have you ever tried to take a nail out of a piece of wood and you couldn't find a hammer or a crowbar? The claw of the hammer and crowbar is what makes a big difference in the effort you make. The difference between having an advantage and leverage is that, leverage allows us to use a compounded force or power to achieve the results we want. Talking through and overcoming victim mentality is a way of building up the leverage towards motivation.

Think of a baseball pitcher lifting his leg towards his chest and leaning back before throwing the ball. He is using his body weight and stance as leverage to compound the force of that ball. Likewise, an archer pulls the bowstring far back before releasing it so that the arrow is propelled further. Can you imagine baseball and archery or many other sports scenarios without these moves? I dragged you through all of this because I wanted to give you the leverage to find the motivation.

We know losing weight is hard and keeping it off is hard too. Regaining the lost weight is every dieter's nightmare and keeping the effort going can be hard. We need something to keep us motivated for the long haul. Here's some advice that seems contradictory. In an earlier section, I had written about how external motivation does not last and can backfire. Just like everything else, there are exceptions. When your external motivation lines up with your internal motivation, and even your introjective motivation, you can achieve so much more than you ever thought you could. This kind of leverage can take you from the motivation that stems from *What's in it for me?* to *What's in it for us?* Below is the last example for this chapter. You will be able to identify the different motivators in this narrative.

I hadn't seen Heloise in about a year, and when I saw her recently, I did a double-take. She had undergone gastric sleeve surgery and looked like a different person. She was diabetic and had been morbidly obese. Over time, she had developed peripheral neuropathy, arthritis in the knees and hips, hypertension and high cholesterol. Every step was painful because there was so much pressure on the knees, and her feet were constantly painful to the point where she could never get restful sleep. Moving around was a burden and she was always out of breath. I could hear her labored breathing from outside a closed door. She even told me that showering was a process. She would have to get into the shower and wait until the pain subsided a little from that exertion, and then start showering. Going to the supermarket was an ordeal too. She had to use those electric shopping scooters, or "fat carts" as she called them. She also needed someone to go with her because she couldn't carry the bags herself. Meanwhile, the diabetic neuropathy became bad enough that she had to have one toe amputated after it became infected. The surgery didn't go well. The surgical site became infected, and she lost two more toes.

At this point, her children and grandkids had to move in and help. She became more helpless and dependent on her family. One day, she looked at her family and thought *"This isn't right. I'm supposed to be able to help them, not the other way around."* Her acknowledgement of the burden to herself and her family, along with the desire to help her family was powerful motivation. After the surgery, she said to me with a big smile, "I can sit on the couch and see part of the seat it in front of my belly. I can walk without pain. I don't have to have someone walk with me down the grocery aisle to get the stuff off the shelves for me. I can move!" She lost over 80 pounds and had been able to get off her cholesterol medicine, her blood pressure medicine and decrease her diabetes medicines.

Some people train for marathons to benefit cancer or walk for multiple sclerosis. They do it not necessarily for themselves, but for a loved one, or for a friend. Even though we say self-motivation or internal motivation is stronger than external motivation, the most powerful form of motivation is rarely just about ourselves. We make changes to be good stewards of our health and our life, but it is also often because we want to be good parents, spouses, or children. It is because we care deeply about the well-being of others who share our lives. When we give of ourselves just because we care, we become part of something much greater than ourselves. This is how we live our lives not in a linear path, but in its entire depth, height, and breadth. When we change our habits because we care, we change our destinies.

4. Comfort Eating

"Emotional illness was a storage disease, and the secret of mental health was to tell the person who hurt you that they hurt you, when they hurt you."
David Viscott

Something very important is often missing from our conversations about weight loss – that is, the painful, emotional experiences leading to weight gain. Numerous books have been written about weight loss, and there are many medications available to suppress appetite, but there is not a lot of guidance about how emotions cause weight gain and how to deal with them. There is plenty of research about whether soda or diet soda makes you gain weight, but not why a person drinks one soda after another, unaware that they are doing it in a mindless way. There are theories about what makes people gain weight and why they struggle to lose weight, yet, for many people, their emotional state may be the true cause of weight gain.

Many articles tell you what to eat, what to avoid, and what to ask your doctor. Some medical weight loss clinics provide counseling on diet, exercise and medications; however, they are rarely equipped to deal with the deeper emotions overwhelming someone and causing them to seek refuge in the comfort of food. Food is a natural source of comfort, because it doesn't criticize or insult; it always welcomes and nourishes.

Emotions and Gaining Weight

At the basic level, weight management can be regarded as the balance between calories consumed and expended. But as we all know, it's never that simple. Behind the calculations and commonsense is a human being with deep emotions. The calculating parts of our brains are interacting with our emotional brains—with one winning over the other at different times.

People gain weight for various reasons, and not everyone gains weight because of their emotions. However, people with Post Traumatic Stress Disorder (PTSD) aren't able to focus on their present habits, because they are troubled with traumatic reminders of their past. They find it difficult to change the coping strategies that have allowed them to survive their psychological trauma. Because food can be comforting during highly stressful periods, binge eating and consistently eating too many calories can lead to weight gain, as well as preventing the shedding of pounds. For some, obesity and weight gain may be a symptom of a mind filled with horrible memories of the past and physical disorders.

There are many forms of trauma. Our childhood homes are typically where many of these events occur. Abuse and neglect have a major effect on an individual's mental health. Violent physical and psychological attacks can also change a person's mental health almost overnight. In addition to dealing with physical disorders such as insomnia, and anxiety, attempts to lose weight may need to address emotional trauma. Some sexual assault victims lose weight, only to regain weight when they hear a compliment because they associate compliments and attractiveness with their former abuse and gaining weight becomes a way of self-preservation and a coping mechanism.

David Viscott, who I quoted to begin this chapter, was a popular psychiatrist in the Los Angeles area during the 1980s and 90s. His work delved into the sources of emotional problems and how they can be remedied through talk therapy and medication. He stated that "Emotional illness was a storage disease." Although Viscott wasn't necessarily talking about obesity but about the emotional burden of pain, anger, and guilt, this can also be applied to weight gain.

In some cases, to survive a cumulative state of distress, people may unintentionally replace it with another storage disorder. When people feel trapped in a seemingly hopeless situation, food often offers an outlet for anxiety—the path of least resistance. People go through these emotions at their own pace. Those who are aware of their emotions learn to reach out for help and are better able to recover from life's events. This is why advice, such as "Just start eating 500 calories less," or "Start exercising," or "Get your doctor to prescribe some medicine," can have the opposite effect of encouraging someone. Instead, it can be perceived as being insensitive.

The secret ingredient to changing our habits is understanding who we are and how we "tick." Research tells us that our motivations are guided by our past experiences[1]. I know this may be the hardest part of your journey toward a healthy lifestyle, but in the end, it's worth it. Because of television shows, celebrities, and news coverage, the stigma of getting mental help for ourselves is starting to go away. One way to address this is to start a weight loss plan while investigating coping mechanisms and help, thus beginning to feel better as you progress.

How Do You Deal with Stress?

Stress is something we deal with, but most of us rarely discuss it with others and typically deal with it through our cache of coping mechanisms. Some of these mechanisms have long histories, going as far back to when we were infants. Everyone copes with stressful situations through their own unique ways. Correlations have been found between drug abuse as a coping mechanism for post-traumatic stress disorder (PTSD[2]). Other severe traumas may result in phobias[3], like agoraphobia and fear of unsafe places, causing some people to rarely leave their home.

Emotional eating may have a link to your past, or it could be as simple as making you feel good. Regardless of where it comes from, we need to know how it affects us, because it can feel overwhelming and hit us from out of nowhere. Craving specific foods, such as junk food or ice cream, is a form of emotional eating. For some of us, these provide relief in a way this is not physically satisfying. As a matter of fact, eating these things may make us feel uncomfortable. This is a type of impulsive eating, when you eat to the point of feeling sick, which can result in feelings of guilt and shame.

Adding to these feelings are the sharp, sometimes unintentional remarks made by friends and family about your weight. If someone taunts you each time you exercise by saying, "So are we trying to compete for Miss Universe?" these words can have a devastating effect. It hurts even more if the people making such comments happen to be someone that you look up to, or if you are a child and it comes from someone that you depend on, like your parents or a role model. Teasing and jokes about weight are thinly cloaked insults and harassment. A friend of mine dealt with people who said these so-called jokes by saying, "It's only funny if both of us are laughing." Her example shows how important it is to stand up against bullies, because it reinforces our determination toward our goals.

Society can be quick to judge and criticize someone for being overweight or obese. There are times when advertisements or careless public comments can make you feel embarrassed and stunned. Remember those plastic surgery billboards along the Interstate? Advertising for cosmetic surgery and weight loss clinics can make you feel that you are somehow not good enough, which is why it's so important to understand when those feelings occur and to redirect our impulses.

Understanding Emotional Eating

Stress, anxiety, and past experiences are a few of the feelings linked to emotional eating. Knowing when these feelings begin to flood and overwhelm you is important. As a coping mechanism, eating can be a way to quiet these feelings and help relieve the discomfort. At the same time, some foods trigger reward and pleasure centers in your brain[4]. This creates a vicious cycle of over-eating or binge eating. To break the cycle, those feelings need to be permitted. Traumatic events require special care, so finding support in a mental health professional may be the best route to take.

These feelings can be subtle and difficult to understand. The "Why?" is not as important as the moment they appear. Recognizing the arrival of an emotion can help us reflect upon our coping mechanisms. Already knuckle-deep in a pint of ice cream? Stop eating and look around to see what triggered you to grab it in the first place. Maybe you're alone that night, or a friend said something earlier in the day that felt mean or spiteful. Was your boss especially hard on you, or did an employee not want to listen? One strategy that some of my patients use, is to ask themselves, "how bad will I feel after I eat all the ice cream?" Knowing they will feel bad, disappointed, or guilty sometimes makes them stop before they go too far. Once they start doing this, they become more and more empowered.

One of the best ways to reflect upon your day can be done in a personal journal. It doesn't have to be eloquent or long. As a matter of fact, using a handful of words to describe the day may reproduce the events that led up to your bad feelings, feelings tucked away until you got home. This allows you to express your emotions and a way to find new strategies to cope with them.

The Difficulty with Trauma

Brenna's story is an example of how we deal with intense emotional trauma. Brenna and her sister were bounced from one foster home to the next when they were teenagers. They had little stability in their lives, yet managed to stay together through it all. They were in their late twenties when Brenna's sister went to work and never came home. She had disappeared.

For the first time, Brenna was completely alone in the world. She felt like she had no one to talk to. No one to give her advice or support. Months went by before Brenna received a phone call from a police officer. They had found a body and positively identified it as her sister, who had been kidnapped, sexually assaulted, and brutally murdered.

While spiraling deeper into depression, Brenna turned to food as her only source of comfort. Not a day went by without her thinking about how she might have been able to prevent her sister's death. Gaining weight and obesity was the least of her worries.

Major Life Events

When I met her, Charlotte was a divorced single mom. While she was married, her husband had been cheating on her. Shortly after their divorce had been finalized, he was quickly remarried, which added to the painful separation. She worked two jobs to make ends meet while taking care of her young son. She was smart and pretty, but also depressed. While she told me her story, it was evident that there had been some emotional abuse in her marriage, and during that time she turned to food.

Coping with the abuse and infidelity through food, she had gained far more weight than she wanted. Right after the divorce, her son was still very young, and she needed a babysitter so that she could go to work. But, now that her son was older, she didn't need a babysitter as much as she used to. Her part time online job was starting to show some promise of consistent extra money. She finally had the time and the means to take care of herself. She spoke with a lot of pain and some anger, but determination was written all over her face. Charlotte understood that her weight gain was from comfort eating. She chose a weight-loss plan knowing it would also address her emotional pain.

Physical Challenges

After quietly dealing with weight issues for many years and not being able to make progress, some people decide to change because of a singular experience. Malcolm Gladwell, the best-selling author and journalist, described a moment like this as a "Tipping Point," when a seemingly simple, everyday event is the reason for dramatic change. This term is usually applied to change occurring at the population level, like epidemics, but it can be applied to individuals as well.

For Ann, that moment came during a flight from Tampa to New York. Traveling alone, she found her seat toward the back of the plane and motioned a flight attendant over. She was having difficulty getting the seatbelt on, so she quietly asked the flight attendant for a seat belt extender. The flight attendant nodded, and went to find one. Somehow, she must have gotten busy and forgotten where Ann was sitting, because as she came walking down the aisle, she held up the seat belt extender, and asked loudly, "Who asked for the seat belt extender?" Ann was absolutely mortified as she raised her hand, feeling the eyes of everyone in that section of the plane. Ann said to me, "My face was burning and I just wanted to die, but at the same time, I knew I was going to do something about it as soon as I got off the plane." This was Ann's tipping point.

Another example is Stephanie, who had planned a vacation for her family and her sister's family to a major theme park in Orlando. They were all very excited to ride the latest roller coaster based on their favorite movie series. The ride was very popular and they stood in line for what seemed like an eternity; people moved at a snail's pace, and the heat and humidity were unbearable, but they finally reached the ride and settled into their seats. Then, the ride operators came over to lower the safety bars, and one said to Stephanie, "I'm sorry ma'am, you'll have to get off. I can't fasten you in completely." She stepped away, biting her lower lip, and stood in front of the remaining crowd. Fighting back the tears, she said to her family, "You go ahead, I'll see you later." She knew then that things were going to change.

I remember Ann, Charlotte, and Stephanie because they each lost 40 to 90 pounds. I am also impressed by how they reacted to the "triggers" that prompted them to take action. And I remember Brenna because she wasn't at the point where she could do anything about her weight. She needed good counseling and support first. Everyone is different, and people are ready for change at different times in their lives.

Mindful Eating

For Charlotte, becoming aware of her emotions and eating mindfully was important in getting her life back on track. When she moved on from the abusive relationship, she first attended to her young son's needs. Once her internet business took off, she felt she had enough stability to use some money she had saved to start a diet program and purchase a gym membership. She also began practicing mindful eating. As she adjusted to her new diet and exercise routine, she used her ability to focus and plan to her advantage to further expand her business and to go back to graduate school. The last time I heard about her, she was in a happy relationship.

Not everyone has these results, because with these success stories come stories of failure, which is why understanding emotional eating is so important. We need to become mindful of what we are eating and understand our body's signals. Feelings of hunger cannot be mixed up with feelings of anxiety, guilt, or shame. Learning about ourselves is part of the journey through life. Mindful eating means paying attention to all the characteristics of the food we are eating, including the smell, taste, and texture. It is a method of eating where you avoid any distractions during your meal, like texting, watching TV, or reading the newspaper.

Pre-planning your meals takes away some of the power of emotional eating, which is almost automatic and a distracted way of eating. If you're feeling hungry, take a moment and think about why before you reach for the pantry door. These are strategies to become a mindful eater. Once you understand the emotional influences of your eating habits, it's time to move on to the external or environmental influences that encourage or reinforce our habits.

5. The Triangle

"As to methods there may be a million and then some, but principles are few. The man who grasps principles can successfully select his own methods. The man who tries methods ignoring principles, is sure to have trouble."

Ralph Waldo Emerson

We have looked at some of the reasons why we quit diets, such as our emotions and motivation. We have also looked at the diseases we could develop if we fail to change our habits. I would consider these to be issues at the individual or micro-level. Now, it's time to look at the bigger picture, or macro-level.

In this chapter, I would like to give you more insight into how we interact with food in our daily lives. To do this, I am borrowing an example from epidemiology, the area of science that looks at how diseases spread. Epidemiology examines the person who gets infected by the disease, the agent that causes the disease, like a bacteria or virus and the physical environment where the infection happens. It has a broad mandate beyond infectious disease to include chronic and occupational diseases. On the next page is a diagram of a triangle[1] used by epidemiologists to describe disease transmission. We can apply this to how we interact with our food and environment and each tip of the triangle has a description in the tables. Along these lines, researchers have been studying how things in our environment, like chemicals, can change how our genes behave without changing our DNA sequence. This process and the research is called epigenetics and cancer is one area being studied and obesity is also an area of interest.

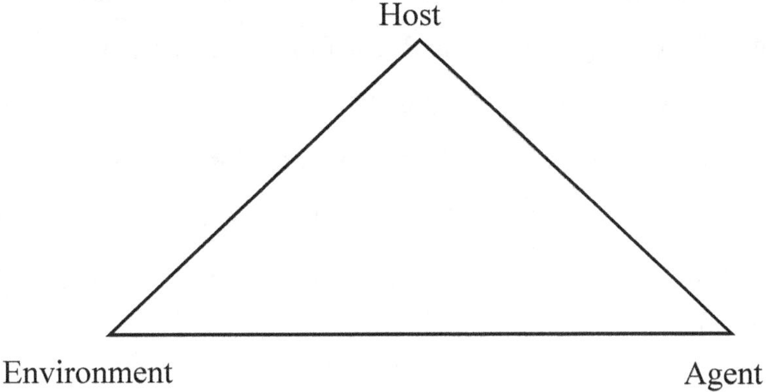

1. We are the host and bear the following characteristics:

• Genetics	• Physical Restrictions
• Height	• Personality
• Skeletal Frame	• Personal Choices
• Hormones	• Habits
• Mental State	• Spirituality

2. The Environment describes the external forces that affect an individual. These are the people, places, and events in a person's life that come and go over time. Some examples of environmental influences are:

• Friends	• Family
• Culture	• Celebrations
• Coworkers	• Relationships
• Work Schedule	• Type of Work
• Stress	• Food Preparer
• Decision Maker	

3. Food is an "agent" found in abundance throughout the developed world. Ready-made meals and fast-food restaurants provide convenience for busy lifestyles. Because of advances in farming and food sciences, our food lasts longer. Global transportation has also contributed to the continuous supply of food in all corners of the world. But, this all comes with a price. How does it impact you?

The World May Be Round, But We Live in a Triangle

The growth of the obesity epidemic can be compared to the spread of infectious diseases. Losing weight involves understanding, accepting, and managing all three components of the triangle. A fad diet addresses the agent—food—one thing, while disregarding everything else, including cost, access, sustainability, and lifestyle.

Best-selling books have investigated the overabundance of food, the food industry, and why it has grown so much over the past 70 years and they are great resources for learning about our food. Food science and agriculture have developed the fastest ways of growing, processing, and selling food. Today, food is modified and preserved to be shipped around the world. In the United States, grocery stores are filled with thousands of choices including many that are not healthy or nutritious.

We tend to overeat in part because food is available in abundance. Laws in some cities around the country have been passed to restrict the selling of certain types of food and drinks such as soda. Placing restrictions on the size of soda addresses one of the components of the triangle and nothing else. Food labels provide great information, yet the large packages don't encourage healthy portions.

The typical adult is the host in this example. Many issues related to the host are beyond our control: age, adult height, race, ethnicity, gender at birth, genetics, who our parents are, and the circumstances we are born into. A young child has no control over what their parents feeds them, but we gain control of our lifestyle, schedules, money, and food choices as we grow older. Our degree of control over other things such as our interpersonal relationships, work and home environments varies depending on the situation. The key is for the host to be aware of the circumstances surrounding their eating habits. Cultural influences are some of the most powerful because they hold the strongest emotional bonds between us and our family and friends. We are social creatures, and food is involved in all our interactions and celebrations.

Cultural Influences

Some types of food are symbolic and integral to holidays and major milestones in our lives. What would a birthday celebration be without cake? Or a wedding? In many cultures, not just America, brides and grooms feed each other cake and champagne in a symbolic gesture of love. There are also many holidays with food traditions of their own.

We could say that food gets power through traditions. Indeed, we could say food is power in many situations. People may be divided along political or religious lines and certain discussions may be taboo, but discussions about good restaurants and good food is always an ice breaker and something that can offer common ground in many instances.

In Asia, a person might take a spoonful of food from a platter and place it on another person's plate in a common gesture to show goodwill, respect, and courtesy. The host often personally serves the guest of honor, and it is customary for the guest to eat everything on their plate in appreciation of the host's kindness. To leave the food uneaten is considered rude.

The gesture of feeding another living being is one of caring and goodwill. Regardless of whether they fly, swim, or walk on two legs or four, a mother feeding her baby symbolizes life. Mahatma Gandhi said, "Where there is love, there is life." I think we can also say that where there is love, most of the time, there is food. But there are times when this expression of love and nurturing turns into dread, fear and resentment.

We may have heard someone say, "I dread going to my grandmother's house because she makes the best brownies and gets upset if I don't eat a lot." We don't want to appear ungrateful and it is easier to go with the flow and take the path of least resistance. Some of us have childhood memories of our mother or grandmother making bread or cookies, and of carefree days when eating was fun and not associated with guilt. Our brains get wired to associate food with love, and when we reject food we feel we are rejecting love. And we don't know how to deal with it gracefully.

For some, this is agonizing. I met a woman who was driven to tears from frustration because she wasn't seeing progress in her weight-loss efforts. She explained that her husband, who loved her dearly, loved sweet foods as much as she did. Despite knowing she was on a diet, he insisted on buying and sharing sweet and decadent food with her. She found it hard to resist, not just because of her sweet tooth, but because she realized that it was his language of love. She was upset that he was sabotaging her effort, but didn't know how to tell him because rejecting the food meant rejecting him.

It's hard enough to resist tasty food, and harder when it is seasoned with love. The struggle is not so much between us and our food but more to do with mutual acceptance, harmony, and the status quo. We need to recognize this struggle and identify where it is coming from to shed a light on the relationships causing the conflict and our own emotions involved when they occur.

Eating Feels Good

Bear with me when I say it's my opinion to think of food as being "an infectious agent," but only when someone is vulnerable to it. Here's an example from when I was waiting for a plane in the airport terminal. One woman was seated drinking a latte from a famous international coffee shop. A second woman walked over and sat down across from her. Noticing the drink, she leaned over and asked, "Where did you get that from? I didn't see it on my way here." The other woman pointed and said, "It's there, next to that restaurant, but it's kind of tucked into the corner." The second woman stood up and said, "Thanks! I **need** my large caramel macchiato, extra shot, extra-whip." The seated woman smiles and replied, "I'll have to try that sometime." After a short wait, the woman returned with her drink. Both exchanged smiles and a few friendly words.

"Transmission" has occurred, and unlike the infectious disease transmission in epidemiology, no one got sick or hurt. As a matter of fact, it made them feel good. The one woman was vulnerable and receptive, yet no one else sitting in the waiting area had the same reaction. Or, they may have been affected by the sight of the cup but were silent. Why was this a bad thing? In general, it's not a matter of good versus bad. The coffee shop is not to blame. They are offering delicious treats for the weary traveler. The individual needs to be conscious of their decision, or else they are susceptible to "food transmission."

But for the individual who struggles with weight, the large caramel macchiato had over 500 calories. That's an entire meal! Maybe, if she was more aware of her surroundings, her emotional state of mind and the calories in the large drink, she could have made a better choice, possibly getting a small with nearly half the calories. Then, she could have reduced the portion while feeling good.

Are You Vulnerable?

In epidemiology, an infectious disease is transmitted when the host is vulnerable. We get infected when we breathe in bacteria or viruses, or eat them in our food. Others get into our bodies through cuts or scrapes in our skin. On the other hand, food is inert, and does not get into our bodies without us eating it. Yet, it tempts us in many ways. In the previous chapter, I pointed out how people eat more than they need when they are stressed or depressed—comfort eating. At times like this, we may gravitate to foods that we were exposed to as children that gives us the temporary comfort that we seek.

On the other hand, you are never susceptible to foods that you don't care for. One example is Sandra, who became a vegetarian because when she was a child, she was repelled by her father's hobby of hunting and the smell of blood from cleaning the animals. Another example is raw clams and oysters. Some people love raw clams and oysters while others can't understand why. The same food is considered a delicacy for some and not for others. Cooking with fish sauce, a flavoring used in Asian cuisine, can be a huge turn-off for some, because it smells rotten to them. So, for tea drinkers sitting in the airport terminal, they were immune to the large latte. It would be nice if we had the ability to be immune and guarded against such breaches, just as we wash our hands to prevent flu transmissions.

We are prone to overeat when we feel hungry. A physical sense of hunger may be real or our body's misinterpretation of thirst or tiredness. Emotional triggers of hunger may include depression, stress, or boredom, such as a long layover or flight delay. Food offers a temporary distraction, and this is when our guard is down, our "immunity" is low and we are vulnerable.

While food is inert, we are tempted by its sight and smell. The temptation grows when there is easy and unlimited access to food. Think about the all-you-can-eat dinners, usually for fundraisers: fish, pancakes, shrimp, and BBQ ribs. Going to all-you-can-eat buffets, free refills on soda, ready to eat meals are other examples. When food is convenient, or of an amazing value with little financial cost to us, we tend to become less restrictive in how much we eat. I have also seen people use this type of reasoning when food is called a "super food" or a type of food that supposedly helps us lose weight, such as pineapple and almonds. Some think that if a little is good, more must be better.

Memories of certain foods can have the same effect. They remind us of good times and we throw caution to the winds. Meals around the time of traditional holidays, especially when they come close together, all add up. We go from home to home, restaurant to restaurant, celebrating with family and friends. In less than two months, we can gain 5% or more of our weight.

The setting in which food is presented can also influence us in significant ways. Researchers followed 150 people[2] over a one-year period to determine how well they performed with their diets depending on their lifestyles. The results showed that when people ate in social settings, such as restaurants and social gatherings, they ate more and strayed from their diets. This implies that we become even more vulnerable to food in abundant quantities and while around other people.

Many of us eat half of our entrée in a restaurant, then bring the rest home in a container. We feel pleasantly satisfied, but not full, and think we have been "good," because we know that the entrée was enough for two meals. The following day, we eat what is in the box and realize that the half portion is quite filling. Yet, at the restaurant, we ate a similar amount, plus a drink and a salad and felt satisfied, but not stuffed. We wonder how we managed to eat that much. This example shows how restaurants and social settings have a way of distorting our perception of portion sizes, catching even the most conscientious dieter off-guard. This has nothing to do with the restaurant's menu or service. Our vulnerability to food in such settings is part of our sociability. We describe someone with a delightful laugh as having an "infectious laugh." Social environments with food could be seen in the same way.

The Big Picture

The ideas presented in this chapter give you a perspective of the "landscape" around you and help you understand the challenges in different situations. Understanding your environment helps to prepare for different life situations. A good example of this is how experienced wilderness hikers would prepare for a journey. First, they select a location, study the terrain, the best time to travel and weather. They make sure they have a good method of communication, and select the appropriate gear, water, and provisions before leaving. This allows them to have a safe and enjoyable experience and prepares them for any nasty surprises. The same is true of weight management, because without a thoughtful plan our weight-loss efforts may be for naught.

A diet doesn't prepare us for social eating, and neither does an exercise wrist band. Depending solely on such things reduces our success because they work in isolation and we don't. We aren't hermits. We are social creatures and celebrate life with our families, friends, and communities. Preparation begins with understanding the triangle, which lets us understand the world around us and how it affects our decisions.

6. Zones of Influence

"We need a witness to our lives. There's a billion people on the planet... I mean, what does any one life really mean? But in a marriage, you're promising to care about everything. The good things, the bad things, the terrible things, the mundane things... all of it, all of the time, every day. You're saying 'Your life will not go unnoticed because I will notice it. Your life will not go un-witnessed because I will be your witness'."

Susan Sarandon's character, Beverly Clark
from "Shall We Dance?"

As we discussed in the last chapter, our environment has a major effect on our diets. It puts macro pressures on our lifestyle and food choices. Fast food restaurants and coffee shops are located in high traffic areas for visibility, access, and profitability. They offer consistency and convenience, taking complete advantage of our fast-paced modern lifestyles.

Our challenge is to make sensible and healthy choices when the options are so plentiful. Lunch at work is a prime example. Your office is possibly located near fast food and sit-down restaurants, making it convenient to step away, take a break, and get lunch. However, your choice was made in the morning to not bring a lunch. Or, if you did, you may leave it there for tomorrow, because someone asked you to go with them.

Your individual choices are also affected by what I call the zones of influence or boundaries, or the micro pressures on our food choices and behaviors. In other words, our decisions about food can be affected by the interpersonal exchanges with the people closest to us, or with those who we cannot avoid interacting with.

What Takes away Our Control?

Zones of influence are greatly dependent on the factors that make up the triangle in our lives. The potential for establishing our zones of influence grows with our level of independence. As we grow older, we have more control over our choices. This was also stated early in the last chapter, so it shouldn't be a surprise here. For parents, their zones of influence change after having children, because they are the ones who plan and prepare the family meals. It would seem that mothers and fathers have a strong ability to establish their zones of influence since they control what their family eats.

This is partly true, but family dynamics can change that balance. Economical and convenient meals are important to middle income families because the parents work, and the families are on a budget. They follow separate schedules for most of the day, only coming together for dinner. Families with school age children are extremely busy, getting tied up with after-school activities and sports. Sometimes, cooking is the last thing on their minds, which is why convenience often wins over healthy home cooking. The abundance of food, food choices, and social norms (who and how you identify with people in general) control your choices, as well as the need to feed the family.

I think that a parent's basic desire is to make sure their family is fed and comfortable. Yet, the needs and preferences of each family member might be different. The meal planner does their best to address all their needs and must often compromise while keeping an eye on the budget.

Relationships Affect Healthy Eating Habits

This is not a book about relationships, but there is no doubt that they play a major role in our lives and influence our diets. Major life events such as a new romance, birth of a child, death, major illnesses, and divorce, all disrupt our lives. It can take a tremendous amount of effort to work through such events when they are associated with deep emotional issues and uncontrollable weight gain is involved. These are times when we are vulnerable to breaches in our zones of influence.

I began this chapter with a quote from the movie, "Shall We Dance." We are social beings and cannot thrive in isolation. We dread living a life that is unwitnessed and forgotten. Marriage and committed relationships involve two people who have promised each other accommodation of the highest order. This means flexing and breaching each other's boundaries.

New relationships are exciting. They involve romance, passion, and fire and couples overlook many differences and habits during this period. After a while, the novelty and excitement abate and life settles in to a routine. For two lives to merge and co-exist successfully in the long term, numerous compromises must be made - for better or for worse. We often see couples who we just know belong together. As couples' zones of influence blur, they adopt each other's mannerisms and may even share similarities in their body habitus. They walk and talk like each other, read each other's minds and finish each other's sentences. They also adopt each other's lifestyles and food habits. Yet, I sometimes meet couples who, while resembling each other in many ways, bitterly complain that they don't have the support to make healthy lifestyle changes together, such as quitting smoking or losing weight. This shows how the blurring of boundaries can become detrimental to our health and weight, and we will see examples below.

Creating Boundaries Is the Key

I like to think of the times, persons, places, and situations affecting our control related to food as very fluid boundaries, or zones of influence. In the ideal world, we would always have 100% control over what we eat. The moment there is a second person in the equation and we plan on eating together, even without sharing the same plate, our zone of influence can shrink to about 50%. Because of love, friendship, and sometimes, simply for the sake of being amicable, we surrender half of our decision-making capacity to someone else. The same could be said of the other person. When our boundaries cross and the zone of influence is breached, we scramble to find common ground. And sometimes, hamburgers end up looking like a good compromise. Over time, this subtle "tug of war" continues until both people admit they have gained too much weight. Then, the cycle of dieting and breaking the diet together begins all over again.

This is where zones of influence and boundaries need to be re-established—to take control over our choices. It's dinner time, and yes, the children need to be fed. But, are you hungry? You had a huge lunch with clients and are about to sit down for dinner with your wife after a long day. Do you need more to eat? For many people, establishing a zone of influence almost becomes an attempt at self-preservation. The obesity epidemic comes from the abundance of food and our lack of control over our choices. Zones of influence are established by anticipating, planning, and setting boundaries. Here are some examples:

- Losing ten pounds two months before Thanksgiving and controlling portions through Thanksgiving, Christmas, and the New Year. Starting a diet the week before a major holiday is doomed to fail. Holidays always come on schedule. Planning ahead gives you an advantage.

- Losing 20 pounds of pregnancy weight over a one-year period before becoming pregnant again. Beginning a diet as you start gaining weight in your second pregnancy is difficult.

- Eating a calorie-controlled breakfast and lunch, because these are the meals you eat by yourself. Then, you have a slightly larger dinner, which you eat with your family. This is a boundary that allows you to take part in your family routine and not feel left out.

- Packing small meals and snacks before you rush through the airport, so you don't have to eat on the run. This is especially helpful if you travel through multiple time zones.

- Looking up restaurant menus and calories prior to eating out. Many restaurants post their nutrition data online, making it easier to make smart decisions.

- Eating only one portion of a restaurant meal and taking the rest home. Guaranteed, if you eat the entire meal, you will feel worse, because you ate too much.

Some Examples You Can Relate with

It's around noon on a weekday. A couple of co-workers walk by. One says, "So what do you want for lunch?" and the other one laughs and replies, "I don't know, but I don't want to have a salad, again." They giggle as they walk away. A short while later, they return with burgers and fries.

Another day, a co-worker pokes her head into my office. "We're ordering from the restaurant down the street. Let me know what you want." I wonder how many times this ritual is repeated before lunch time in workplaces all over the country. After the rush of the morning, lunch is a chance for a break, a chance to build camaraderie, and to gear up again for the afternoon. After lunch, everyone settles down with full stomachs. A similar ritual is likely repeated at dinner time—each and every day.

Over time, ordering food at work becomes a habit, one that is hard to break. It's probably harder to break up with your lunch buddy than to break up with your hair dresser. It is awkward to tell your lunch partner that you don't want to order food with them anymore. If you really want to break up with your hair dresser, you can always find another hair salon. But, it's hard to avoid your cubicle neighbor without looking like a spoilsport or appearing cheap, when you sit next to them every day.

To me, these interactions are less about food than they are about friendship, caring, empathy, team building, bonding, and love. Therein lies the problem. Sharing meals is about your relationship with others; love and affection, compassion and social bonding with others, which are all necessary for healthy human interactions. We need to love and feel loved. Food has been central to this human need since the dawn of time. It creates and strengthens relationships. But, if we look at the evolution of our social eating habits, food was never as abundant as it is today, which makes it harder to establish boundaries. We may not be able to create a perfect boundary, but it can be done.

Some people need to reclaim their zone of influence by breaking away. Here is what happened with Cynthia and Gregory, who have been married for a long time. They have had the good fortune of being successful in business. Their children are all grown up and moved out.

Life has been good, and they love each other. They are open about their feelings for each other and are very affectionate. They did almost everything together, including traveling and eating out a lot. Over time, they gained weight, but now it was affecting Gregory's health. Cynthia was still in good health, but she hated how the extra weight made her look and feel.

They agreed to work together to lose weight, and both did well during the first few weeks. They reminded each other when they strayed from the diet. There was a little friendly competition between the two of them, as well as a lot of encouragement. However, as is often the case, Gregory was losing weight faster than Cynthia.

At first, there was some joking back and forth, of how Cynthia had a "bad day" at work that prevented her from focusing on the diet. But then, Gregory started slowing down, and Cynthia seemed to be slowing down even more, with no explanation. Then one day, Gregory admitted that there had been trouble for several weeks. Cynthia greatly resented that Gregory was losing weight faster than she was. And she was very vocal about it and felt that Gregory wasn't being fair to her. The arguments got to be so bad that Gregory purposely started eating more food to avoid losing weight.

There was a very good reason why he lost weight and she didn't, even though they had most meals together, shopped together, and exercised together. They basically mirrored each other in their weight loss and exercise plan. Cynthia couldn't understand why Gregory would lose more weight, if they walked the same number of miles, and spent the same amount of time on the treadmill. The reason why Gregory was losing weight faster with the same amount of exercise was because he had the advantage of having a higher metabolic rate. Gregory is 6' 2", and Cynthia is about 5' 1" (Metabolic rates will be discussed later in the book, for now, the focus is on relationships).

About a year later, Gregory was not just back at square one, but had gained an additional 25 pounds and suffered a heart attack. He had also lost his old job but did manage to find another one. This was when Gregory decided to go on a medical weight loss program without telling Cynthia. The new job enabled him to attend the program during breaks, and essentially enabled him to work on his own weight loss goals without Cynthia knowing about it. He also carefully planned his lunch and dinner, which he always had at work so that the only meal he had to have with Cynthia was dinner. He did not feel good about doing these things behind her back, but at least he had reclaimed his zone of influence.

Sometimes the interaction between two people can result in one person enabling the other without either one of them realizing it. Terry had been a member of a local weight-loss support group for three years and she had never missed a meeting. Sometimes she lost weight and other times she gained. Terry explained to me that she would come back from her meetings and happily announce her loss of three pounds to her husband, then say, "I have been starving myself all week, and craving pizza." Then, her husband Phil would say, "I think you have earned it. When do you want to go?"

Another week, Terry comes home dejected. Phil knows what happened, and asks, "Are you ok?" Terry says, "I can't believe I gained 5 pounds this week." Phil says, "I don't understand it. I know you've been good." Feeling defeated, Terry responds, "This program isn't working for me. What's the use? I don't want to think about it tonight. I'm just hungry right now, and I don't feel like cooking. Phil says, "I know honey, it's just going to stress you out even more. Let's go to our favorite restaurant and

have some wine and pasta. You can always get back on track next week."
Terry is the stronger personality in the relationship, but she has no real
sense of her zones of influence. Phil adores his wife and can't bear to see
her unhappy. He cares more about comforting her than supporting her
efforts. In the process of pleasing her and keeping the peace, he has
become the soothsayer and enabler, and in doing so, steps over Terry's
boundaries. Unlike Gregory, Terry hasn't woken up to the fact that she
needs to establish her own zones of influence.

The next story is from someone who used to be in sales in a very
fast-paced and high-pressure industry. His employer had a strong focus on
building relationships with clients which meant that his time on the job
meant a lot of entertaining, eating, and drinking with clients and
prospective clients[1]. It got to the point where, in his own words, he was
"drinking like a fish", and he gained a lot of weight. He decided he had to
quit drinking when his family life began to suffer, and he was no longer
happy with his job. Up to this point, he could not even think about being
able to do his job without drinking. The business depended on
relationships, and relationships are best built around food and drink. Food
and drink were the tools of the trade. To let go of these tools was
unthinkable.

He felt that the more he could drink, the better he could influence
his customers' purchases. He writes, "I laugh now. How naive could I be
to think that customers' buying decisions were based on my ability to
drink shots?" He decided that he didn't need to drink to do his job, but his
clients could, if they wanted to. He started to take clients out for lunch
instead of dinner until he lost any urgent desire to drink. When he did
resume taking them to dinners, he cleverly instructed the bar tenders to
bring him club soda each time he asked for a vodka club. He started going

to the gym very early in the morning. Ultimately, he lost weight, regained his family life and satisfaction with his work. He had established his zones of influence on his own terms, by controlling the timing, the type of meals, and even instructing the restaurant staff. In addition, as we discussed in the chapter on motivation, he used all four forms of motivation, and because of his dedication to his family, he has a better chance for success in the long run.

7. To Count or Not to Count

Two young fish swimming along, and they happen to meet an older fish swimming the other way who nods at them and says "morning, boys. How's the water?" And the two, young fish swim on for a bit, and then eventually one of them looks over at the other and goes "What the hell is water?"

David Foster Wallace - This is Water -
Value of Self Awareness

The last two chapters described who and what affects your weight loss plan. Even for the most motivated individual, when lifestyles, habits, and partners are not aligned, there is no diet that can help you lose weight in the long term by itself. Our environment and interpersonal relationships have a huge effect on how we eat. Learning how to control these areas through creating boundaries is not easy and requires motivation, support, and persistence. Once they are created, your ability to count and control the number of calories you take in is much more manageable. Many people dread counting calories even though the equation is seemingly simple:

Calories/Energy in – Calories/Energy out = Weight loss or gain

There are 3,500 calories in a pound of fat and we say more physical activity, exercise, and fewer calories consumed will result in weight loss. Let's say you eat 500 fewer calories a day, then after 7 days you will have lost one pound. This seems simple, but if you are asked to eat 500 calories less, the question is, less than what? Is it less that the 2000 calories listed on the nutrition labels, or 500 less than what we ate yesterday? As we know, all calories are not created equally and there are variations in how our bodies process food. Hormones and water weight may also vary the numbers on your scales.

It may be harder for some people to lose weight than others, because their metabolism is different. Body mass, age, and gender play a part in the equation that affects our Basal Metabolic Rate (BMR), which we will discuss later. For now, let's concentrate on calories.

Basically, calories are a unit of measurement, a way for scientist to explain how food becomes energy. A calorie is the amount of energy needed to raise 1 gram of water 1 degree Celsius. It is very small, and that's all the science we need to know—food becomes energy. And, our bodies use energy, whether we are resting or moving and exercising.

Olympic athletes, like Michael Phelps, are said to eat almost 5,000 calories in a day while training and competing. Their bodies convert the food to energy quickly and efficiently. Dietary changes for high performance athletes are sometimes difficult when decreasing their training regimen, because they are used to eating a higher number of calories.

Counting Is Not Difficult, It's Second Nature

Diets require a reduction in the number of calories per day, so we can begin to burn the stored calories throughout our bodies. Some people get distressed at the idea of counting calories, portions, or carbohydrates. They say "I don't have the time to do it," and "it's too hard," or "I don't do counting." The reality is, counting is inherent to our thinking, as natural as walking, and a part of our physical make-up. It's instinctive and essential to survival.

We learn to calculate very young. There are some videos of cute toddlers caught on baby cams who wait until their parents turn off the lights, wait for a couple of minutes, then start climbing out of their cribs. When we cross a busy road, we calculate our walking speed and the speed of the oncoming car to see if we can get across to the other side before the car hits us. In our minds, we visualize the intersection of the trajectory of the car's path and ours. We figure we'll be ok, if we can get beyond that point before the car reaches that spot.

We became the dominant species because of our cognitive abilities, one of which is the ability to make calculations. Calculative skills require concentration, memory, and attention. But, in our hectic, modern life, we have a hard time remembering what we ate two days ago, which is why a journal is so important. I once helped two couples lose weight at the same time and one couple decided that they didn't need to keep a journal. The other couple documented everything, even their exercise. The first couple accomplished so much more in the same amount of time than the second couple. By the way, the couple who lost more weight drove three times the distance to check in each week, giving you an idea of how much motivation and determination matters.

How to Document What You Eat

Trying to remember the days we stuck to our plan, ate fewer calories, and ended up with a caloric deficit is nearly impossible unless we write it down somewhere. It is also difficult to remember the days we go over our limits. That's why writing down or keeping track of what you eat is important. It can be as simple or as detailed as you wish. Some find it easier to document at the end at the end of the day, others write things down as they go along. Some write the type and amount of food and the calories consumed. Others make a note of the time of the meal, such as breakfast, lunch, dinner, and snacks. Beverages should be noted as well.

Writing this down after each meal isn't easy, but there are phone apps and gadgets to help count calories. Some can be expensive or require a monthly fee; however, if that fits your lifestyle, then they may be a big help. The key is to find the one that best fits your personality and lifestyle; one that can help you keep track every day. Among my patients, those who kept track of their calories always had an advantage over those who did not.

While there is an abundance of nutritional information online, as well as some great calorie calculators for smartphones, reading labels on food packaging is also important. There is useful information in the labels, especially when you track carbohydrates. These labels will also help you see the difference between high- and low-calorie options. Also, start to learn how big a serving is for everything you eat: meat, fruit, veggies, and starches. Here is a list of calories per serving for common foods[1] based on the American Dietetic Association recommendations *(note that meat is measured after being cooked)*:

Vegetables contain 25 calories and 5 grams of carbohydrate. One serving equals:

- ½ C of cooked vegetables (carrots, broccoli, zucchini, cabbage, etc.)
- 1 C of raw vegetables or salad greens
- ½ C of vegetable juice

Fat-Free and Very Low-Fat Milk contain 90 calories per serving. One serving equals:

- 1C milk, fat-free or 1% fat
- ¾ C yogurt, plain nonfat or low-fat
- 1C yogurt, artificially sweetened

Very Lean Protein choices have 35 calories and 1 gram of fat per serving. One serving equals:

- 1 oz. of turkey breast or chicken breast, skin removed
- 1 oz. of fish fillet (flounder, sole, scrod, cod, etc.)
- 1 oz. of canned tuna in water
- 1 oz. of shellfish (clams, lobster, scallop, shrimp)
- ¾ C of cottage cheese, nonfat or low-fat
- 2 egg whites
- ¼ C of egg substitute
- 1 oz. fat-free cheese
- ½ C of beans, cooked (black beans, kidney, chick peas, or lentils): count as 1 starch/bread and 1 very lean protein

Fruits contain 15 grams of carbohydrates and 60 calories. One serving equals:

- 1 small apple, banana, orange, nectarine
- 1 medium fresh peach
- 1 kiwi
- ½ grapefruit
- ½ mango
- 1 C of fresh berries (strawberries, raspberries, or blueberries)
- 1 C of fresh melon cubes

- 1 / 8 of a honeydew melon

- 4 oz. of unsweetened juice

- 4 tsp of jelly or jam

Lean Protein choices have 55 calories and 2–3 grams of fat per serving. One serving equals:

- 1 oz. chicken—dark meat, skin removed

- 1 oz. turkey—dark meat, skin removed

- 1 oz. salmon, swordfish, herring

- 1 oz. lean beef (flank steak, London broil, tenderloin, roast beef) *

- 1 oz. veal, roast or lean chop*

- 1 oz. lamb, roast or lean chop*

- 1 oz. pork, tenderloin or fresh ham*

- 1 oz. low-fat cheese (with 3 g or less of fat per ounce)

- 1 oz. low-fat luncheon meats (with 3 g or less of fat per ounce)

- ¼ C 4.5% fat cottage cheese

- 2 medium sardines

  * Limit to 1–2 times per week

Medium-Fat Proteins have 75 calories and 5 grams of fat per serving. One serving equals:

- 1 oz beef (any prime cut), corned beef, ground beef**

- 1 oz pork chop

- 1 whole egg (medium)**

- 1 oz mozzarella cheese

- ¼ C riccotta cheese

** Choose these very infrequently

Starches contain 15 grams of carbohydrate and 80 calories per serving. One serving equals:

- 1 slice of bread (white, pumpernickel, whole wheat, rye)
- 2 slices of reduced-calorie or "lite" bread
- ¼ (1 oz.) bagel (varies)
- ½ English muffin
- ½ hamburger bun
- ¾ C cold cereal
- 1⁄3 C rice, brown or white, cooked
- 1⁄3 C barley or couscous, cooked
- 1⁄3 C legumes (dried beans, peas, or lentils), cooked
- ½ C pasta, cooked
- ½ C bulger, cooked
- ½ C corn, sweet potato, or green peas
- 3 oz. baked sweet or white potato
- ¾ oz. pretzel
- 3 C of popcorn, hot air popped or microwave (80% light)

Fats contain 45 calories and 5 grams of fat per serving. One serving equals:

- 1 tsp. of oil (vegetable, corn, canola, olive, etc.)
- 1 tsp. of butter
- 1 tsp. stick margarine
- 1 tsp. of mayonnaise
- 1 tbsp. of reduced-fat margarine or mayonnaise
- 1 tbsp. of salad dressing
- 1 tbsp. of cream cheese

- 2 tbsp. of lite cream cheese
- 1/8th of an avocado
- 8 large black olives
- 10 large pimento stuffed green olives
- 1 slice of bacon

Servings Versus Portions

The National Heart Lung and Blood Institute (NHLBI) states, "Did you know that a portion is different than a serving of food? A portion is the amount of food (big or small) you choose to eat. A serving is a *measured* amount of food or drink." As you can see from the list above, servings in this small sample of familiar foods have a set number of calories. Basic servings follow these guidelines. Think of *calories* being the smallest unit of measurement, like an inch, *servings* being a slightly larger unit of measurement, like a foot, and *portions* being what we ultimately choose to eat, like a yard. The serving considers the type of food and quantity, and the number of calories vary among the food groups.

Commercially labeled foods also display the calories per serving, and the number of servings in a package. However, the definition of servings on the Food exchange list and those on food packages can differ. For example, the serving size on the label of a box of cereal is calculated by dividing the package in half or more. Although servings technically have a defined number of calories per food group, the servings in a box of cereal are equally measured. These should be called portions, not servings, but the food industry is allowed to do this, and sometimes, it is for convenience, so we must work within the parameters that are set for us. The same is true for recipes. The serving size on recipes often reflect a portion rather than the strict NHLBI definition of a serving. So, if we are cooking for ourselves, the food exchange will be useful, and when we are cooking or eating pre-packaged foods, we would need to look at the nutrition labels or the recipe. As mentioned earlier, a portion is the amount of food you choose to eat. It can have one or more servings in it. But we usually don't eat cereal by itself. Adding milk to cereal will now add some protein and possibly fats, depending on the type of milk. As you can see, we need to be careful when reading labels and stick to the basics of looking at the calories, as well as recognizing the language used by food companies.

Portion Control

The problem with portion control is that calories can add up very quickly. A 300-calorie frozen dinner can be eaten in about four or five mouthfuls. Six chicken nuggets may add up to 300 calories. This is why some people have a hard time with portion control, whether it's fast food (you want fries with that?) or sit-down meals (entrée and sides) at a restaurant. For merchants, they are a business and they're in it to make money. And, we want value—lots of it. So, the amount of food served must justify the amount of money charged. When we eat restaurant food, we are actually getting our money's worth. There are usually two-to-three meal portions for the price of one at most restaurants. And, if we were to eat all of that in one sitting each time we go out, we would most certainly gain weight.

We have better control of portions when we cook at home. One way to understand portions is to start with understanding servings. If you cut a 10-ounce flank steak from the supermarket and cut it into equal pieces this is 10 servings, which look a little more than a single bite. If you were planning on eating the entire steak, then count on 550 calories. Half of this steak is 225 calories. The same can be said of pasta. Typically, one box of pasta is a pound, or 16 ounces. I suggest dividing up the box into four-ounce portions. Now, you can see that one quarter of the box is about five servings, equal to 400 calories. Cut that in half and you have a generous number of carbs to fuel your next workout.

The idea is to hold the amount of food in your hands, see it with your eyes, and learn what a healthy portion looks like. Because, if you think about it, eating an entire steak with pasta is nearly a meal and a half on their own. Add to this the appetizer, salad, and drinks and you have two meals. Because it can become complicated, some of us need quick and easy measurements and may prefer to use a visual guide[2] to portions (see diagram on next page).

It is said that what gets measured gets done. Calculating and counting go side by side with planning. Once you pay attention to what you are eating, then you can plan on what you need to feel full. The Okinawan centenarians said, "Eat only until you are eight – tenths full." This is excellent advice. When we eat, our stomach sends a signal to our brains as it begins to get full, the satiety signal. It takes about 20 minutes for the brain to recognize this signal. So, if we eat fast, we don't allow time for this signal to occur, and when it does, it is already too late. Therefore, you will have better success if you slow down and enjoy the meal over at least 20 minutes, and importantly, pre-plan your portions. Combine this with keeping a journal and you are quickly establishing control over your meals. Some have brushed off the advice on portions and later regretted it.

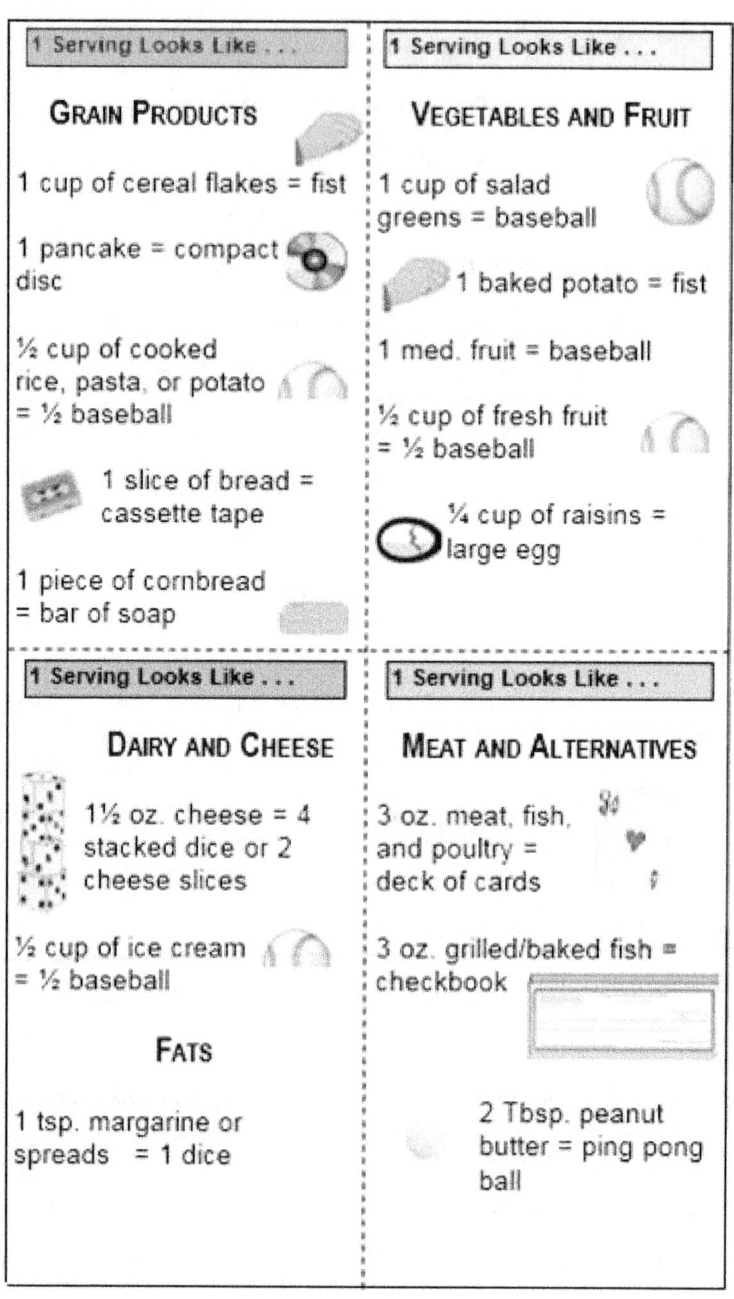

Portion distortion is a real problem and has been for a long time. Restaurants meals and food packaging have changed tremendously over the years to make people feel like they are getting value for their money, when in fact they are getting too much. But, when we think about it, going to a restaurant and leaving hungry is not a pleasant experience either. They would rather you take food home than feel hungry. Carbonated soft drinks have increased in size, too. During the '50s, a bottle of cola was only 7 ounces. Today, you have a choice of 16, 20, and 24 ounces or a 2-liter bottle—filled with high-fructose corn syrup. Just like the triangle and zones of influence, portion distortion is something to be very aware of. There is the expression, "Our eyes are bigger than our stomachs." but it is amazing how our stomachs manage to stretch to keep up with our eyes. Understanding how much a serving of food looks like can counteract the effects of portion distortion and keeps you on track toward your goals.

Read the Labels

Food labels describe the ingredients, nutritional information, and sometimes the health benefits. These labels appear on almost all food, as mandated by the federal government. There are a few exceptions, one of which is alcohol, which we will address in a later chapter. Labels are there to help us understand what's in our food. Processed foods have very complex labeling because of the many ingredients used to preserve, color, and make the food taste good. Frozen vegetables and fruits have simple labels. I highly encourage you to look at the ingredients if you want to be more aware of what you are eating. Use the Internet to research some of the common ones. For now, let's look at how to read the nutrition label. One thing to remember is that the labels are calculated based on the assumption that everyone eats 2000 calories a day, which is just not true, but it is still used as a reference. Also, the calculations are approximate, and companies are only required to be within 20% of the actual number.

For foods with lots of ingredients, you will have to depend upon their numbers, while foods with few ingredients can be checked against our list above. These labels and smartphone applications make it easy to see how many calories are in what you are eating.

Beginning at the top, we see what a serving constitutes, the servings per container along with the corresponding calories per serving. As I have stated, the "servings" on the package are not always the same as the servings given to us by the NHLBI, and sometimes should be considered portions. The nutrition information that follows on the label is based on that label's serving size, so we need to be aware of this when making our meals.

Please read them and enter the information (total calories you eat) into your journal. Labels also describe the food groups and how much is in each group: fats, sodium (salt), carbs, and proteins. Fats affect the heart and are listed at the top.

Nutrition Facts
Servings
Amount Per Serving
Calories
% Daily Value*
Total Fat
Saturated Fat
Monounsaturated Fat
Polyunsaturated Fat
Trans Fat
Cholesterol
Sodium
Potassium
Total Carbohydrate
Fiber
Sugars
Protein
Vitamin A
Vitamin C
Calcium
Iron
*Based on a 2,000-calorie diet, your values may be different. Values may not be 100% accurate and have not been evaluated professionally or by the US FDA.

They are broken down between saturated and unsaturated fats. Too much saturated fat can clog your arteries. Cholesterol and sodium are next and can also affect a person's heart and blood pressure. The government labeling system requires these three components of food to be listed first.

Carbohydrates appear in the middle. Understanding the types of carbs you eat is as important as the amount (grams) in each serving. Carbs have subcategories, *sugars, fiber,* and sometimes, *sugar alcohols.* Carbs that are absorbed into the blood from the intestine give us energy, and extra carbs become fat. Fiber is a carb that stays in the intestine and does not go into the blood. Therefore, it is not counted towards your calorie intake, and it is good for your digestive system. Sugars are carbs that get absorbed quickly and sent throughout the body. Excess sugar is converted into fat and stored for a time when you need it. Sugar alcohols[2] are neither sugar nor alcohol and are used as thickening agents and sweeteners. They do not contribute to our calorie intake, that is, our net carb intake. This is how eating foods with high fiber content, such as whole grains help us reduce our net carb intake.

Proteins are listed after carbs and are important for growth and tissue repair. Their digestive process is different from carbs and they can suppress hunger better, thus the popularity of high protein or low-carb diets. Now that we have reviewed the ubiquitous nutrition label, it's time to demystify and decode the food we are eating to learn what happens after we eat our food.

8. Decoding Food: Digestion and Storage

"Let food be thy medicine, and medicine be thy food."

Hippocrates

In the last chapter, we discussed what's in the food that we are about to eat. Now, we will discuss what happens after we have eaten the food, how it is digested, absorbed, and when we stockpile too much of it.

A question I am asked by people going on diets is whether they will be hungry when they reduce their total calories for the day. This is an important concern and the answer is that it depends on the composition and frequency of the meals. Understanding how our body deals with the food we eat, in other words, demystifying and decoding our food helps us choose the types of food that will help suppress hunger, stabilize blood sugar, and promote weight loss.

Digestion followed by absorption—a complex balance of mechanical and chemical processes—breaks down and moves food throughout the body. As food is broken down into smaller pieces, nutrients are absorbed into our body mainly through the small intestine. When we understand how different types of food get absorbed into the bloodstream and distributed among the cells, we can better manage our weight.

At the Cellular Level

The macronutrients from food provide the cells in your body with vital nutrients for energy or to repair damage to the cell. Each step of the digestion and absorption process breaks carbohydrates, proteins, and fat down into their simplest forms. Carbohydrates are sugars, starches, and fiber. Proteins are composed of long chains of amino acids. Finally, fats are long chains of lipids made of fatty acids and monoglycerides.

The starches we eat, such as pasta or rice, are long chains of sugars that the body breaks down into glucose (a process called glycolysis), the simplest form of sugar, so small that it can easily pass through the cell walls. Carbohydrates provide a quick source of fuel for the body to use and extra carbs are stored as glycogen and fat.

Proteins are long, complex chains of amino acids. They are the building blocks of your cells. These large molecules require more steps than simple carbs to break the chemical bonds holding them together, so they can be absorbed into the body.

Fats also need more time and enzymes to break them down into lipids in the small intestine. Once absorbed, these lipids are formed into triglycerides and are used as energy by cells or stored in fat cells. Our bodies are very good at absorbing and storing fat.

Now that we know a little more about the food we are eating, let's take a more detailed look at how these macronutrients are used by our bodies and why we need to be more conscious of which ones we eat.

Carbohydrates

I have a refrigerator magnet that says, "Life is unpredictable, eat dessert first!" Since the time of our ancestors, our bodies have been programmed for survival. Glucose is our body's most basic source of energy. When our blood sugar levels are low, we may feel hungry, or have trouble concentrating, experience some dizziness, sweating and heart palpitations. Low levels of blood sugar can also affect our mood. The term "hangry" is used for a person who is angry because they are hungry, and it's in the dictionary. In extreme cases of very low blood sugar levels, called hypoglycemia, people may lose consciousness.

Our bodies understand that when energy levels are low, it should use the type of food that is easiest to digest—sugar and carbohydrates—to produce glucose. In other words, our bodies will "Eat dessert first!" and use simple sugars as an easy fix for a quick recovery. People with diabetes know how powerful a glass of orange juice or glucose tablets can be to help recover from low blood sugar, or hypoglycemia. The result can be immediate and dramatic. The digestion of simple carbs and sugars begin in the mouth by the salivary amylase enzyme. There are a lot of carbs in a multi-course meal with a drink, appetizer, bread, salad, entrée, and dessert. Our bodies don't care whether we eat dessert at the beginning or the end of the meal. It will absorb simple sugars before other nutrients.

With increased portion sizes, we eat more than our bodies need. We are left with more unused carbohydrates at the end of each day than ever before. These are stored as glycogen in the liver and smaller amounts throughout the body. This is our back-up supply of energy when we need it for a "rainy day." If there still more carbs, they are stored as fat.

The body uses glycogen before fat. But, with so much food being available, instead of using our existing fat supply, we continuously add more carbs which settle around our waists and our internal organs as fat, because true to form, our bodies simply keep using the new carbs first and the stored fat goes untouched. And, as our society becomes more sedentary, we burn fewer calories than when people were more physically active.

If we want to start using stored fat, we must stop tempting it with what it loves to use the most—sugars and simple carbohydrates. Once the carbs and sugars are used up, it will start to use fat as a main energy source. Eating less carbs activates our body's need to use stored fat. The idea of low carb diets is to break down the stored fat. But, to get to the fat reserves, the body must first burn through glycogen which is like the gatekeeper that our bodies must deal with before breaking down the fat. The liver stores enough glycogen for about 24 hours of activity. Once glycogen is gone, the body starts breaking down fat and the true process of losing fat begins. While avoiding carbohydrates for a week or so can jump start your diet, permanently avoiding carbohydrates is not recommended.

Complex Carbohydrates: Fiber, Fruits, and Vegetables

When we think of carbohydrates, we tend to think of foods such as sugar, white bread, white rice, potatoes, and pasta first. These are simple carbohydrates because they are easily digested. Complex carbohydrates, such as lentils and whole grains have fiber that passes through your digestive system, promoting good colon health, while making you feel more full when eating. Vegetables are carbohydrates as well, but they have lower amounts of carbs, especially leafy green vegetables, per serving.

Fiber acts like a sponge, absorbing water, increasing the volume of your stool, and softening it to prevent constipation and promote regular bowel movements. Fiber comes in soluble and non-soluble forms. They remain in the intestine and do not pass into the bloodstream. By remaining in the stomach and intestine, it increases the volume of the contents, making us feel full for a longer time. Fiber may also prevent cholesterol levels from rising by trapping it in the intestine and preventing it from entering the blood. Some people on low carb diets keep their net carbohydrate intake low (usually around 25-50 grams) by the calculation below. It is the net carbs which directly contribute to our energy supply and weight gain or loss. Since fiber stays in the intestine and passes through the body without entering the bloodstream, they are not counted towards net carb intake. Sugar alcohol, as mentioned in the previous chapter, does not contribute to energy and can also be subtracted.

Net carbs = Total carbs – (fiber + sugar alcohol).

For example, 10 gms net carbs = 20 gms total carbs – (5gms fiber + 5gms sugar alcohol).

A common complaint of people on low-to-no-carb diets is constipation. As they become constipated, they notice that they are losing weight and urinating more. The reason is, when people eliminate all carbohydrates from their diet, there is water loss from lack of dietary fiber. The "sponge" that has been absorbing water and holding it in the intestine, giving stool a softer consistency, is no longer there. The body responds to lack of water by trying to conserve as much water as possible, but it is extremely important for people who use this approach to stay hydrated, and some may benefit from over the counter fiber products, such as psyllium husk.

Vegetables are healthy carbohydrates with multiple health benefits. Is a vegetarian lifestyle healthier than a non-vegetarian lifestyle? In a large-scale study[1] with over 70,000 participants, researchers looked at dietary patterns of non-vegetarians, semi-vegetarians, pesco-vegetarians (those who eat fish), lacto-ovo-vegetarians (those who eat dairy and eggs), and strict vegetarians. Non-vegetarians had a higher average body mass index, consumed more fat and calories, than their non-meat-eating counterparts.

For vegetarians, losing weight can sometimes become a challenge to suppress hunger, use up existing carbs without adding more, and maintain adequate nutrients. When trying to prevent hunger while losing weight, strict vegetarians who avoid eggs and dairy use soy, quinoa, and some other soy products as sources of complete, or near complete proteins that can compare with animal protein. Other sources of protein from vegetables come mixed with carbohydrates, such as beans, or mixed with fats, such as nuts, and ounce for ounce, they contain fewer grams of protein than animal proteins.

Restricting carbohydrate intake causes the body to use up existing carbohydrates in the body including glycogen and start breaking down fat after 4 to 5 days. After fat is broken down and used for energy, a by-product called ketones are formed and are ultimately passed in the urine. This is called ketosis and is the basis for ketogenic diets. When ketones appear in the urine, their presence can be detected by litmus testing, because the acidic nature of ketones will turn the litmus paper pink. Although not the most accurate indicator of fat loss, it is a simple, indirect test that can be done at home. Ketosis should not be mistaken with ketoacidosis, a potentially dangerous condition that can occur in diabetes when there is not enough insulin.

Juicing vegetables is a quick way of getting several servings of vegetables and nutrients in a single portion. This can be convenient for people with busy schedules, but the number of calories and carbohydrates still matter. Some smoothies deliver 300 calories or more in a small container and may contain 15 to 25 carbohydrates. Also, the process of juicing can drastically reduce the fiber content that we would have benefitted from by eating whole fruits and vegetables. If you enjoy smoothies, I suggest looking at the nutrition label and picking those with a higher fiber content.

Some people underestimate fruits and vegetables and their carb content. Chloe wondered why she wasn't losing weight as steadily as she should. She said she had done well on a low-carb diet at first, but then decided to rely heavily on a vegetarian diet after she became bored with the food choices. That marked the time when she stopped losing weight. She admitted that she was not measuring the servings and portions for vegetables because she thought vegetables were "free" as in being free of calories, and that she could eat as much as she wanted to. Vegetables contain calories and they are carbs, some healthier than others. Green vegetables will give you about 5 grams of carbs per serving, and starchy vegetables like corn, potatoes, and beans will give you much more. By not differentiating the types of vegetables and not controlling portions, she was undermining her own efforts. There are many restaurants that offer colorful and large portions of salad. They also sometimes post the calories. You may be surprised to see that it is not unusual for these salads to have close to 1000 calories. Portions always matter.

Fats: Lipids and Fatty Acids

Fat has several important functions, as a source of energy when needed, as cholesterol to form steroids, neurons, and sex hormones. It also helps absorb the important fat-soluble vitamins, A, D, E, and K that are important for vision, skin, strong bones, and blood clotting. It can provide energy through the break down process of lipolysis; however, in our society, this doesn't happen easily. Excess fat is like the relative that we have always been meaning to call, but never got around to it because life happens, and we get distracted. The body "forgets" about the fat when we continue to give it carbohydrates.

Among proteins, red meat has the highest amount of saturated fat. This type of fat stays solid at room temperature, such as the fat in bacon, or a well-marbled piece of steak. When we consume them in large quantities over time, our cholesterol level rises, including the bad cholesterol (LDL cholesterol) and clog our arteries, causing poor circulation in our legs, and can lead to heart attacks or strokes.

Trans fats are partially dehydrogenated vegetable oils and are more harmful to health than saturated or unsaturated fats. Historically, they were developed in the 1900s from soybean oil during a buttermilk shortage. Trans fats are cheap to make and easy to use. They are useful for packaged baked products and make them last longer. The Centers for Disease Control and Prevention estimates that up to 20,000 heart attacks a year could be prevented by avoiding trans fats. Today, many companies have drastically reduced or eliminated them from their products, but some companies still use trans fats. It's important that we read the labels on processed foods to look for trans fats. Partially hydrogenated fats on a label are trans fats and if they are listed, they should not be within the first several items, where they would be considered a major ingredient and probably much of the calories and cholesterol. It's best to avoid them all together if possible.

The fat found in fish and nuts is different from other fats, because they contain polyunsaturated and monounsaturated fats and are much healthier. While all fats should be eaten in moderation, mono- and polyunsaturated fats can benefit heart health. When following a diet low in carbs, it's also a good habit to focus on proteins and oils rich in these fats, avoiding the ones heavy in saturated fats.

Oils come in different varieties such as olive oil, vegetable oil, sesame, peanut, grape seed, etc., and more are becoming available for cooking every day. They provide around 100-120 calories per tablespoon and are considered healthier than saturated fats. Coconut oil is considered a saturated fat and should be used in moderation. Fat from fish, nuts, and avocadoes are considered the healthiest. Trans fats are considered the worst, and the rest are in between.

Proteins: Amino Acids

Proteins have many important functions such as providing amino acids to form building blocks for muscles, fighting infections, repairing damaged tissues, and serving as a source of energy. The body can synthesize many of these amino acids except for nine that humans cannot produce and must be obtained from food. These are called the essential amino acids. Animal proteins are considered complete because they contain all nine essential amino acids. Most plant proteins are considered incomplete, but products such as soy, quinoa, seiten, Quorn, and hempseed are considered complete or near complete proteins. For instance, similar to animal proteins, soy contains 9 grams of protein per ounce and no carbohydrates. The typical recommendation for low carb diets is 0.8 to 1.0 grams of protein per kg of body weight per day.

Proteins are important throughout our lives. To get an idea of the function of proteins, let's look at some extreme examples. In infants under the age of 1 year, protein deficiency causes swelling of the abdomen and the legs. These children become lethargic and weak. They have anemia, because there is not enough protein to form iron in the blood (hemoglobin carries oxygen to the cells), and they may even have heart failure. They are also prone to infections because of their lowered immunity. This condition is called Kwashiorkor.

Muscle is the type of organ which we either "use it or lose it." Inactivity causes muscles to waste away and activity through exercise develops stronger muscles. The muscles then become the biggest user of energy in our bodies from fat, hence people who are more muscular and exercise can eat more without gaining additional weight. In older adults, a condition called sarcopenia occurs when muscles waste away, causing weakness and fragility. This can lead to falls and hip fractures, because the muscles that stabilize our joints are not strong enough to maintain our posture. Some people with muscle wasting may be not look underweight and still have muscle weakness, because the reduced muscle mass is masked by an increase in their body fat, either from overconsumption of carbs, from inactivity, or both. In fact, some may look obese and yet have very little muscle mass, and this is called sarcopenic obesity.

Excess protein can be stored as glycogen and fat and later converted back to glucose in a process called gluconeogenesis (gluco-glucose or sugar, neo-new, genesis-creation, meaning, the creation of glucose from a new source). The bottom line is, when consumed in excess, carbohydrates and proteins can become fat mass. Moderation is truly the key to maintaining good health and a normal weight.

Glycemic Index

Something rarely discussed in fad diets is the glycemic index, typically regarded as something important for people living with diabetes, but has value for the rest of us as well. The Merck Manual has a good description of how the glycemic index works. Pure sugar (glucose) has an index of 100. This means sugar is very easy to digest and absorb into the blood very quickly. As the blood sugar rises, insulin is released, like the bellhop at a nice hotel receiving new arrivals and escorts the blood sugar into the tissues. And because this is done so efficiently, the blood sugar level drops quickly. If it drops too low, we experience sweating, palpitations, and dizziness.

You can see how foods that are quickly digested and absorbed make your blood glucose go up and down like a yo-yo, and foods that are slowly digested do not. If foods that are easily digested make you feel hungry faster, then slowly digested foods would make you feel fuller longer. This is the principle behind using foods to manage your blood glucose and your hunger level. Foods that are quickly digested include processed foods like sugar and white bread. Processing removes fiber that naturally resists and slows the digestion process. Foods that are slowly digested include whole grains, legumes, animal proteins, and plant proteins. As you can see, most of these are sold in their natural state, ready for the grill or eaten raw.

The glycemic index can be manipulated by pairing high and low glycemic index foods together to reduce the impact of high glycemic index foods and suppress hunger for a longer period. Here is a visual example about how foods have staying power. Think about how long it takes to chew steak (protein). We know that if we don't chew it long enough, we might choke on it. Now, think about how quickly you can chew a muffin (carb) before swallowing. Of course, the steak takes longer to chew, and it takes longer to digest in the stomach, while the muffin crumbles in your mouth. The protein will "stay" with you longer and can hold you until your next meal. A key to weight loss is to select the best types of food that stop hunger for a longer period with smaller servings. The steak and muffin example is only for visual impact, since not all carbs crumble like a muffin and protein shakes don't have to be chewed at all, but you get the point. I typically recommend three portion-controlled low carb meals, and two small measured snacks for the times when you feel like having one.

We switch gears a bit for the next chapter. You'll notice that some popular magazines include a full page of pictures of several celebrities arranged side by side along with captions and comments about the clothing style. The pictures are cropped, and they appear to be of similar height and weight, but in real life, we know that their heights may range, for instance, from 5'2 to 6'0. With the help of coaches, diets, and exercise, the celebrities manage to develop a certain proportion and silhouette. In the next chapter, we will review what normal proportions and body composition should be as well as our energy use based on our body size.

9. Some Important Numbers to Understand

"Life is so much brighter when we focus on what truly matters to us."

Author unknown

There is a point when our bodies suffer from the added stress of extra weight. Each additional pound places more stress on our ankles, knees, hips, heart, and other parts of our bodies. A good example is the force on your knees when you walk. If every step on level ground at a regular pace requires extra effort, the effort increases even more when you walk up several flights of stairs. Regardless of your weight, this is the effects of gravity on your body. But, the extra mass requires the heart to work much harder to circulate your blood.

Our heart is the engine that keeps blood moving through our bodies. No one would dream of putting the engine from a micro-car, like a Smart® car, into a large truck and expect it to perform the same, or last very long. Even though they are very complex, cars are much easier to repair than the human body. Their worn-out parts can be easily replaced. Not so in humans.

Your Body-by the Numbers

We don't have spare parts, so the longer we can make our body structures last, the better off we are. We can better maintain our body by understanding some numbers to manage our weight successfully.

Body mass index (BMI) – Tells you about your proportions, whether you have a lean or broad outline. In other words, your overall shape.

Fat percent – Our bodies are made of different tissues and fat tissue is what we are trying to lose. Not only does fat build up around our waist and thighs, but it also surrounds many of our internal organs.

Basal metabolic rate (BMR) – Calculates how much energy your body's "engine" needs when it is "idling" (resting and sleeping) over a 24-hour period.

These are described in detail below. There are other measurements of our body composition such as lean mass, muscle mass, and water weight, but we will focus on these three because they can be readily measured through tables (BMI), online calculators (BMR), and calipers (fat percent). Some scales and electronic gadgets can provide these numbers and body composition analyzers are available in some gyms.

We can certainly lose weight without ever knowing these numbers, but having this knowledge helps give clarity to the journey toward a healthy weight. These measurements describe a global view of your body and provide good guidance.

Body Mass Index (BMI)

This gives us a specific number and a range. It is an imperfect measurement, because it doesn't account for our body frame, muscle mass, or the state of our health. BMI simply describes your body's overall proportions and what your general silhouette looks like. Based on height, it gives us a range for our lowest and highest ideal weight and where we currently fall. Keep in mind that "out of proportion" doesn't necessarily equate to being out of physical condition or bad health. Nevertheless, because it is a simple measurement only requiring a scale and a measuring tape, it is a good place to start. In the charts below, find your height on the left side, then find your weight in one of the corresponding columns (there are many online BMI calculators available to use, too). Your weight is in the column indicating your BMI[1].

BMI	19	20	21	22	23	24	25	26	27	28	29	30	31	32	33	34	35	36
Height (Inches)								**Weight (Pounds)**										
60	97	102	107	112	118	123	128	133	138	143	148	153	158	163	168	174	179	184
61	100	106	111	116	122	127	132	137	143	148	153	158	164	169	174	180	185	190
62	104	109	115	120	126	131	136	142	147	153	158	164	169	175	180	186	191	196
63	207	113	118	124	130	135	141	146	152	158	163	169	175	180	186	191	197	203
64	110	116	122	128	134	140	145	151	157	163	169	174	180	186	192	197	204	209
65	114	120	126	132	138	144	150	156	162	168	174	180	186	192	198	204	210	216
66	118	124	130	136	142	148	155	161	167	173	179	186	192	198	204	210	216	223
67	121	127	134	140	146	153	159	166	172	178	185	191	198	204	211	217	223	230
68	125	131	138	144	151	158	164	171	177	184	190	197	203	210	216	223	230	236
69	128	135	142	149	155	162	169	176	182	189	196	203	209	216	223	230	236	243
70	132	139	146	153	160	167	174	181	188	195	202	209	216	222	229	236	243	250
71	136	143	150	157	165	172	179	186	193	200	208	215	222	229	236	243	250	257
72	140	147	154	162	169	177	184	191	199	206	213	221	228	235	242	250	258	265
73	144	151	159	166	174	182	189	197	204	212	219	227	235	242	250	257	265	272
74	148	155	163	171	179	186	194	202	210	218	225	233	241	249	256	264	272	280
75	152	160	168	176	184	192	200	208	216	224	232	240	248	256	264	272	279	287

BMI	37	38	39	40	41	42	43	44	45	46	47	48	49	50	51	52	53	54
Height (Inches)								Weight (Pounds)										
60	189	194	199	204	209	215	220	225	230	235	240	245	250	255	261	266	271	276
61	195	201	206	211	217	222	227	232	238	243	248	254	289	264	269	275	280	285
62	202	207	213	218	224	229	235	240	246	251	256	262	267	273	278	284	289	295
63	208	214	220	225	231	237	242	248	254	259	265	270	278	282	287	293	299	304
64	215	221	227	232	238	244	250	256	262	267	273	279	285	291	296	302	308	314
65	222	228	234	240	246	252	258	264	270	276	282	288	294	300	306	312	318	324
66	229	235	241	247	253	260	266	272	278	284	291	297	303	309	315	322	328	334
67	236	242	249	255	261	268	274	280	287	293	299	306	312	319	325	331	338	344
68	243	249	256	262	269	276	282	289	295	302	308	315	322	328	335	341	348	354
69	250	257	263	270	277	284	291	297	304	311	318	324	331	338	345	351	358	365
70	257	264	271	278	285	292	299	306	313	320	327	334	341	348	355	362	369	376
71	265	272	279	286	293	301	308	315	322	329	338	343	351	358	365	372	376	386
72	272	279	287	294	302	309	316	324	331	338	346	353	361	368	375	383	390	397
73	280	288	295	302	310	318	325	333	340	348	355	363	371	378	386	393	401	408
74	287	295	303	311	319	326	334	342	350	358	365	373	381	389	396	404	412	420
75	295	303	311	319	327	335	343	351	359	367	375	383	391	399	407	415	423	431

For instance, if you are 5 feet and 9 inches tall, your weight should ideally range between 125 pounds and 160 pounds, corresponding to a BMI of 18.5 to 24.5. This range is considered healthy, meaning that the engine and the gears that make our body run are matched to our size. Within this weight range our knees can comfortably support our bodies, and our heart can pump enough energy rich blood through our circulatory system, regardless of whether we are sleeping, sitting, or running.

An obese man and an athletic man may have the same height, weight, and BMI, but have very different body tissue compositions and look very different. The obese man will have a larger waist circumference, and the athletic man will be broader at the chest, and more muscular around the arms and legs. This simple BMI calculation does not take body tissue composition into consideration. For instance, a man who is 6 feet tall and weighs 225 pounds has a body mass index of 30.5 regardless of whether he has more fat than muscle or vice versa. And, he would be considered obese. There are some body builders who were denied health insurance or were forced to pay a higher insurance premium simply because of their higher BMI.

Fat Percentage

There are two types of body fat, subcutaneous and visceral. Subcutaneous fat is the fat under our skin and is probably what bothers people the most, certainly before they lose weight, and often, even after they have lost weight and achieved their goal. People feel happy as they start losing weight, because their back and knee pain improves. They start feeling back in control as their blood sugar and blood pressure start to settle. Yet, many people, especially those who have lost a large amount of weight, are disappointed when they are left with loose folds of "skin" around their arms and abdomens. Commercial advertisements show before and after pictures of people who have lost large amounts of weight. They don't necessarily show pictures of these folds. The advertisements urge people to get in shape for the summer, promoting a "beach body," and it is disheartening when the reality is not always what the ads promised. I have met many people who lost close to 100 pounds and end up feeling defeated after working hard for many months. This is probably the most emotionally charged issue for this chapter.

People develop these "skin folds" because they worked hard and lost weight, and they should be very proud of themselves. But, it is understandable to want to have a more streamlined appearance. I have met people who lost a lot of weight either by dieting and exercise, or in combination with bariatric surgery. I have also met people who, much to my dismay, decided to put the weight back on because they hated the loose folds so much, and felt that all their efforts were wasted. And others went through a second surgery to reduce the loose folds.

What are these loose folds, and are they inevitable? After the age of 30, we accumulate fat, especially around our middles. Pick up a fold around your abdomen and see how it feels. Does it feel very thin, like the skin over the back of your hand? If so, that is indeed, loose skin. But if there is a thicker roll between your fingers, then, that is subcutaneous fat covered by skin. The vast majority of people, even many celebrities have a roll of varying sizes.

It is hard for someone who has worked so hard to lose weight to feel that they now need to lose fat. The results can be dramatic when people go back for surgery to remove this fat and some skin. It is an expensive procedure and may not be covered by health insurance. I advise people who have a lot of weight to lose to put a little bit of money aside each week or month as they lose weight, so that they know that if they feel the need to have skin folds removed, they will have some funds ready. This also reminds us that it is better to start losing weight early than to wait until the skin is too stretched.

Before we call fat the bad guy, I want to say that it is excess fat, especially fat inside our abdomen that is harmful. A reasonable amount of overall fat, that is less than 30% for women and less than 25% for men is considered average[2]. Fat gives our faces softness and youthfulness, forms the basis for hormones, and insulates our bodies.

Visceral fat, even though it is not visible, is more harmful than subcutaneous fat. It surrounds our internal organs such as the liver and intestines, and lines the inside of our blood vessels, including the delicate vessels that supply our hearts and brains. Visceral fat can harden over time, causing problems, especially for the heart.

Subcutaneous and visceral fat are something we have in common with other mammalian species, such as rats that are typically used in research labs. Researchers have shown that rats with greater visceral fat developed insulin resistance (a risk of diabetes). When the fat was removed, their bodies started using insulin as effectively as young rats. Moreover, research[3] has shown a correlation between body mass index, visceral fat, and developing type 2 diabetes. The study involved over 3,000 people throughout the United States. The researchers used CT scans to measure the visceral and subcutaneous fat.

How does one measure visceral fat without a CT scan? The waist circumference[4] is a good measurement. It is measured just above the hip bones while breathing out and can be done on your own. A waist circumference of greater than 40 inches for men, and greater than 35 inches for women, places them at higher risk for diabetes and heart problems.

Special scales can estimate total fat mass using a method called bioelectrical impedance. How it works is very simple. It sends a small current of electricity through your body from one foot on the scale to the other and measures the time it took. Fat is a slower conductor of electricity than muscle. There are also handheld versions of this machine, and some are a combination of scales and handles for a more accurate reading. But, a simple manual caliper can be purchased for less than $10.00 and do a fairly decent job to measure fat percentage. It's not how much the tool costs, but what you do with the information that ultimately makes the difference.

You may know someone who lost weight and hated the subcutaneous fat, but saw an improvement in their blood sugar level as their insulin resistance went down. Losing visceral fat causes weight loss and shrinks the waistline. Logically, this means there is less internal support, less visceral fat (and some muscle) to prop up the subcutaneous fat, making it hang down in loose folds. As far as I am concerned, this should be a tremendous motivating factor showing the power of our own capabilities. Our appreciation for our own strengths should grow when we know what to focus on.

Basal Metabolic Rate (BMR)

When people talk about having a "slow metabolism," this is often what they are talking about, but some may not relate it accurately to their body mass. Your basal metabolic rate (BMR) represents the number of calories you burn at rest over a 24-hour period. This is like the gasoline that a car uses while idling at a traffic light. When adjusted for physical activity, BMR forms the baseline number for how many calories you will burn during an entire day. This is the basic concept behind the "energy in – energy out" equation. Unlike cars, our body's engine cannot be turned on and off completely with a key. Our bodies are still working even as we sleep. The simple idea is that, if we don't move around much at all and keep eating more calories than our bodies' BMR, over time, we would gain weight. On the other hand, if we eat just around our BMR requirements and move extra, over time, we should lose weight.

However, BMR is influenced by certain factors. Men have the advantage of having a higher BMR, and BMR declines about 2% every decade in adulthood[5]. Also, the more we weigh, the higher the BMR, because there is simply more mass to maintain and move, just like it takes more energy to heat and cool a large house than a small house.

Here is another example. I have a small SUV that runs at 22 miles per gallon. My friend, Annabelle, has a big truck that runs at 9 miles per gallon. If we both drove 100 miles, my SUV will use 4.5 gallons of fuel, and hers would need 11.1 gallons for the same distance, almost three times the amount. In an earlier chapter, I described a couple where the husband was losing weight faster than the wife, making her unhappy. This is because as a larger person, he used up more energy during exercise. Whether it is a human or a car, greater mass simply needs more energy to move. Some people who are overweight or obese mistakenly believe that they cannot lose weight because their "metabolism is slow." The truth is, the greater the body mass, the higher the BMR. Men have daily calorie needs typically around 2000 calories per day and women may average around 1500. To find a more accurate number that best represents your BMR, there are many calculators to choose from online, such as this one at https://www.active.com/fitness/calculators/calories[6]. I suggest taking an average of 3, since results may differ around 100 calories. Some apps calculate your BMR plus your daily activities for you. By staying close to these calorie numbers and adding exercise, you can increase your energy expenditure above your energy intake to effectively lose weight. Many people find this calculation helpful.

Using Numbers as Boundaries

Picture frames exist to train our eyes on the picture or painting within the borders of the frame. The same is true when we know our ideal boundaries and numbers, because we can focus sharply on what matters. We deviate less from our plan and these numbers make it is easier to correct any excursions beyond the boundaries. Knowing our bodies' framework gives us the same freedom as when we close our doors at night, defining and controlling the boundary between private and public spaces, so that we can close our eyes and sleep in peace.

There is not much we can do to modify our gender or age. However, there is one thing we can change. When we exercise, and our muscles contract and relax, the action pumps blood rich with oxygen through our blood vessels. Just like the fuel that runs a car, the nutrients, including fat, are used to supply the oxygen to the exercising muscles. As the muscle develops, it continues to use the "fuel," whether we are active or at rest. Although it will not double or triple your metabolic rate, people with more muscle mass can eat more food and not accumulate fat. Maintaining muscle mass means exercising regularly. It's much easier for someone who is in shape or has more muscle mass to lose weight quickly and keep it off.

10. Exercise

"Those who think that they have no time for bodily exercise, will sooner or later have to find time for illness."

Edward Stanley

There are countless exercise programs and gyms that are structured creatively to be fun and effective. Yet, we still hear or read discussions about which exercise is best for losing weight. Any exercise is always better than no exercise, but it can feel like a chore if it doesn't fit our lifestyle or if we don't enjoy it. Some people may have a medical condition that prevents them from participating in strenuous exercise programs. For a person who can't take part in exercise, cross-fit, or run long distances, suggesting that they "just get moving" can be plain annoying.

Exercise needs to be tailored to our physical abilities, especially when you are just beginning to exercise. The Centers for Disease Control and Prevention (CDC) recommends combining both acrobic exercise with strength training[1], and several options from which to choose. Aerobic activity increases your heart rate and strength training works the muscle groups in your entire body. Beginners may want to start with 150 minutes of walking and two days of muscle strengthening. The 150 minutes could be 30 minutes of walking a day spread over five days.

How you want to look and feel is also important when choosing the types of exercise. Lifting weights, cross-fit, running, swimming, or doing only cardio, or a mix of it all can get you in great shape and allows you to sculpt your body at the same time. Exercise maintains and builds muscle, which, in turn, helps burn more fat. A combination of diet and exercise burns fat quicker and makes you feel better at the same time.

Exercise doesn't come naturally to all people and some simply dread it. I can remember one woman, let's call her Jenn, who wanted to lose weight without exercising. She was willing to stay on a diet, but dead set against any form of exercise at all although she had no physical limitation. She wanted assurance that she would lose weight without exercising. I said, "Sure, you'll lose weight, but you may not like the way you look." She wasn't very happy to hear this, but it's how our bodies tend to work, as described below.

The Body: A Highly Efficient Energy Storage System

Let's start with an example. When we get home from grocery shopping, we pack the fridge with perishables and the pantry with dry goods. As we use up the groceries, we sometimes forget what is at the back of the fridge or pantry. We could say that the forgotten food in the back is like the stored fat in our bodies. Fat cells throughout the body, the liver, and muscles store different forms of energy. When we limit our calories, our body starts looking in our body storage areas to see where it can get the calories to make up for the energy we need each day, which is our BMR plus our physical activities. As the stored energy is used up, we lose weight. Our bodies use what is readily available, starting with simple carbohydrates and glycogen, and then fat. Some muscle mass will be lost too, in a process called gluconeogenesis, but if we include proteins in our diets and exercise, the muscle is protected. People who only diet and don't exercise can develop flabbiness in their arms, legs, and abdomens, because their muscle mass wasn't protected, and they lose lean as well as fat mass.

Muscle strength and mass are important, especially as we grow older. We have all seen older people who have a hard time getting up from a chair or from bed. It's not always because they have arthritis or back pain, but from muscle weakness. As I mentioned in the last chapter, when people become less active with age, their muscle can be replaced by fat, in a condition called sarcopenia. An extreme example of muscle loss is when someone suffers from a stroke and becomes paralyzed. Not being able to use the muscle leads to muscle wasting called atrophy. Lower levels of testosterone in men can also affect muscle mass.

There are two types of muscles in our body, voluntary and involuntary muscles. The muscles inside our bodies, such as the muscles of the heart, around our arteries, and within our intestines are not under our control. When we get stomach cramps, those are our involuntary muscles contracting. On the other hand, we control the voluntary muscles on the exterior of our bodies, such as our arms, legs, abdomens, and backs. They are also called command muscles, which means they respond to us, their commander. If we have them at our command, why should we not use them to our advantage?

Our Body's "Thermostat"

Our body has special mechanisms in place to keep us stable and comfortable. When it is cold, we shiver to maintain our core temperature at 98.6F. The rapid contraction and relaxation of muscles produces heat[2]. When we are warm, our blood vessels receive signals to dilate, allowing more blood to flow through and disperse heat through sweating.

These are some of the things that our body does to keep all our systems running in harmony and to adapt to changes in our environment. A similar mechanism takes place when we gain weight. Our body tries to keep our weight stable, but over time, as our weight creeps up, it accepts a higher level of body weight as the new "normal" weight. This process is called energy homeostasis, whereby our body adapts to the higher energy needs of a greater body mass. When we lose weight, the body tries to again keep things stable by preventing us from losing weight, and when it lasts longer than we would like, some call it "plateau." I describe it as the body "resting" for a bit while assessing our new needs[3]. At this point, intensifying your exercise routine and persisting with your diet is your best plan of action to continue losing weight. This is seen even after people have reached their goal weight and for some people, it may feel like a twisted game of "limbo" where hard work leads to more hard work. If people regain some of the weight back, it is not necessarily a failure, but emphasizes the importance of exercise.

A Lesson from the Car Dealership

When you walk into a car dealership, every car has a sticker in its window. On that sticker is a gas pump icon showing the gas mileage for highway and local roads. The highway gas mileage is always higher. For example, a car might get 25 miles to the gallon on local roads and 32 miles on the highway. Now, if this is your car and you're driving mostly on the highway, you're getting more miles for each gallon of gas. The car is running more efficiently and sipping the gas more slowly, so you get more miles for your money.

When the same car is driven on local roads, there are multiple traffic lights, corners and stop signs. Some stop lights last several minutes, while you wait, and your car idles without moving an inch. Frequent stops mean the car must slow down, and brake, then speed up again over short distances. Before reaching a cruising speed, the car uses extra gas to gain the momentum it needs.

If you're a person trying to lose weight, you want to think in terms of highway mileage and local driving. Highway mileage occurs when you have exercised to the point where you can make your body go long distances effortlessly. You have just transformed yourself into an efficient machine. It sips fuel! Except, the fuel is fat and now you are burning it sparingly. Exercise is good, but sometimes it can have unintended results.

Susie wanted to lose about forty pounds. She started with a diet but didn't plan on exercising. After the first couple of weeks, she wanted to lose weight faster, so she started walking. She had realized that dieting without exercise was too slow. She walked about 30 minutes every other day and started feeling better and steadily lost weight. To mix up her exercise routine, she started riding a bicycle. She enjoyed this so much that she rode further and further until she was riding over 100 miles a week! However, as the miles increased, she began to lose weight at a slower rate, until she remained at a plateau. She was in great health, but she wasn't happy.

Energy efficiency is what you want for long distance running or biking. But, when you are trying to lose weight, inefficiency is your friend. It's not that you can't lose weight while you are doing long-distance training, it's just that it will take longer. Also, some people may eat more than they should after exercising, because they felt they have burnt enough calories to not have to worry about eating as much as they want. This was the case with Susie. Also, remember the discussion in the previous section about how the body resists changes in our weight thermostat. Susie was up against all these challenges.

When Susie started biking less and mixing in other forms of exercise like weights, she did start losing fat again. The exercise sessions should be short enough and challenging enough that it requires extra effort. When the level of effort to move a mass is varied over short periods of time, whether it is a car or our bodies, the extra effort made to regain lost momentum expends additional energy.

Another story is from Mila, who was a runner in her twenties. She loved the endorphin rush and the wind in her face when she ran. She could run for miles every day, but she couldn't lose enough fat. She was training for a marathon and trying to lose weight at the same time and couldn't make any progress. While she was making a conscious decision to lose weight, her body was trying to stabilize her. Also, marathon training required that she eat enough carbs to sustain her energy levels making it difficult to go back and forth between lower and higher carb levels.

She decided to mix in cross-fit while running a bit less. After her first week of reduced miles, she lost one pound from fat mass. The following week, she lost 2.8 pounds of fat mass, which encouraged her even more to continue with cross-fit training. And the subsequent week, she lost another 0.5 pounds of fat mass.

High Intensity Means You Need to Work

Many people would like to work out regularly but don't have the time to do so. Recently, high intensity interval training (HIIT)[4] has become popular among people who have limited time to exercise but wanted maximum results. It basically forces you to act like a car driving around town, because of the frequent periods of brief rest between high intensity sets. The difference is in HIIT workouts, you need to go from 0 to 90 when the light turns green. I would imagine you would get a ticket for that in the city.

A HIIT workout forces you to perform at or above 80% of your maximum effort for each interval, each set, resting in between enough for your heart rate to slow down a little. You can see the difference between distance training and stop and go. Your heart is the engine that pushes oxygen and nutrients to the cells. It must keep up with the demands of the bursts of energy. It's much more strenuous for it to start up after each pause, while distance training has momentum.

Another advantage of HIIT over distance training is the focus on all the muscles, not just your legs. The routines are designed to engage large and small muscle groups throughout your body. These workouts tone your muscles and burn away the subcutaneous fat around them.

Increasing the amount of work performed by your muscles requires more oxygen and calories. Studies on HIIT have shown an increase in metabolic rates while resting—after the workout. This calorie burn continues after the workout, up to 15% more, so you can burn calories while resting. If you want to lose weight quickly, consider a workout plan involving HIIT. Consult your doctor first to see if you can. People with heart conditions, poor circulation, or other disorders may not be able to take part in HIIT.

Which Exercise Is Better for You?

There is a debate about whether cardio or strength training is better for weight loss. To answer this question, let's look at people who do each type of exercise regularly. The Olympic athlete is at their peak performance and their best physical shape. Running and sprinting are pure cardio sports. The bodies of these athletes are perfectly streamlined, with long, lean muscles and a relatively low body fat percentage. When standing at the starting line, their body shapes are so similar, regardless of their nationality, they could almost fit into the same mold. Body shape changes and muscles develop in response to the type of sport. Swimmers develop strong shoulders, arms and abdomens. Cyclists and skaters and skiers develop great lower body strength and muscle. Most of us won't become Olympians but we can tailor our exercise pattern to shape our bodies.

On the other hand, weight lifting is a fine example where the emphasis is on consistent strength and resistance training. These athletes have muscular chests, arms, abdomens and legs which add to their overall shape and bulk. Many of them would be considered obese by the standard BMI calculator, even though they are in excellent health (some runners would be considered underweight by the calculator).

These examples show how we can redefine our body shape as we lose weight by picking between cardio (aerobic exercise and cardio are almost interchangeable), or strength training. Cardio is the better exercise for losing overall weight and slimming down, but strength training defines and increases muscle bulk, especially in men. Aerobic exercise involves moving your own body mass and moving mass burns energy.

With that being said, actual results may vary and when two people exercise together, one of them may be disappointed. The more mass there is to move, the greater the energy used and the greater the weight loss, therefore people with larger builds tend to have a somewhat easier time losing larger amounts of weight.

Here's an example using dogs instead of people, just for fun. River, the Weimaraner, and Shelby, the Jack Russell terrier, (both girls) go for a walk together. River lopes along with long legs and Shelby's little legs move rapidly in quick little steps. If they walked the same distance, who would burn more energy per pound? The answer, would be Shelby. But River would have burned more overall energy because she has many times more mass. So, if the scale tells them that River lost more weight than Shelby, she would be disappointed because she had to work harder and lose less weight. This is similar to the example of Cynthia and Gregory in the chapter on Zones of Influence. The question of cardio versus strength training has also been studied by researchers at Duke University[5] and they recommend a combination of cardio (aerobic) exercise and strength training as the best way to lose weight.

If you are neither an athlete nor inclined to join a gym, how hard will it be to lose weight? For Dale, a financial challenge turned out to be a blessing in disguise. Several years ago, Dale and Patty found themselves in more debt than they cared to have. After discussing their options, they decided to sell one of their cars to help pay the debt. This helped tremendously, but now there was a different problem. Patty's work shift started around 3:00 am while Dale worked from 9:00 am to 5:00 pm and they commuted in opposite directions. Because of the early hours, they decided that Patty would use the car, which left Dale with no transportation. There were people who he could have asked for a ride, but Dale did not want to feel obligated to anyone. Instead, he picked up a bicycle from the thrift store. The thought of riding a bicycle approximately fifty miles a day was intimidating, but he had already made his decision. He packed a change of clothing and set out early in the morning. He picked a route that would let him avoid heavy traffic and identified bus shelters where he could stop in case of thunderstorms. Over the next two years he logged over 5000 miles, went through two bicycles and paid off the debt. They had also saved enough money to purchase a new car.

On a drive along his old route, he pointed out things that he had discovered during the two years. Sometimes, he would stop at a small park to see the wildlife. He also found short cuts that not too many people knew about. He says he was in the best shape of his life during those years and kind of missed the ride. Once he bought the second car, he felt the weight creeping up and felt sluggish and uncomfortable. He was now in his sixties and retired. He picked up a different exercise habit and spent a few dollars on a jump rope. When the sun cools off in the evening, he can be seen jumping rope under his carport.

Going back to Jenn, my example of someone who doesn't want to exercise, she will lose weight from burning fat and unfortunately, muscle. The journey toward her goal will be slower than everyone else and she may feel tired from the effort. Plus, she'll be a candidate for regaining much of it back, especially if she wanders from her diet. People like Jenn and others, for various reasons, get frustrated and want to quicken the pace of their weight loss using medications and supplements. These are typically prescribed by physicians and require frequent monitoring. Nowadays, there are more choices in medications, but they are not the magic pills that we would like to have. Not only that, we are unique individuals and we respond differently to medications. In the next chapter, we will discuss medications that affect our weight.

11. Medications and Weight

"Whether you think you can or you think you can't, you're right."
Henry Ford

In this chapter, I address prescription medications used for weight loss, as well as other commonly used medications which can affect our weight. Several Food and Drug Agency (FDA) approved prescription medications used for weight loss are in the form of appetite suppressants. People are surprised when I say, "You know that appetite suppressants won't make you lose weight, right?" Their typical response is, "What do you mean?"

Many appetite suppressants are designed to simply suppress appetite—not to make you lose weight—unless you work with them. The appetite suppressant works only if you actually cut back on calories and exercise. It works through a chemical signal telling your brain that you are not hungry. The use of an appetite suppressant requires you to play an active role in losing weight. Think of it as an assistant, a very small one inside your head, telling you that you don't need to eat very much because you feel full. If you miss the cue and continue eating, you will fail to lose weight. The purpose of the appetite suppressant is simply to give you an *opportunity to train your brain* to regulate your food intake. When that cue is missed, we run the risk of using the appetite suppressant and still struggling to lose weight. While in some cases, this might be because the type of medication was not the best fit, in many cases, it is because of misunderstanding of how the medication works.

When appetite suppressants are not used correctly, they give a false sense of security leading to frustration and disappointment. A useful analogy is when some people with diabetes feel that a normal or near normal blood glucose level is a signal to eat without regard to portions and calories. People with diabetes have a challenge like those trying to lose weight, where they both need to actively manage their calories. Nowadays, there are many excellent medications for various conditions, but depending on how we use them, they may be our friends or foes. Insulin, which is both produced by our bodies, (except for people with type 1 diabetes), and available as a drug for diabetes, is a good example.

The Special Case of Diabetes

In 2004, scientists discovered that cells acted differently in obese mice than in mice of normal weight. When a cell was bombarded with too many nutrients, a structure called the endoplasmic reticulum, which generates energy, sent signals to insulin receptors to shut off the supply[1]. When this happened, the obese mice developed diabetes. This gave scientists an insight into the relationship between obesity and diabetes which they called "insulin resistance."

Ten years later, scientists from the University of Texas ran an experiment on mice to see what happened when they were given very high levels of insulin. Even as their blood glucose level was being regulated, the mice gained weight[2].

These two studies make us think about what happens when we eat too much food and receive too much insulin at the same time. A recent article[3] reviewed several studies where the body weights of people receiving basal insulin were compared to diabetes medications called glucagon-like peptide 1 (GLP-1) receptor agonists. These studies showed across the board that insulin is associated with various degrees of weight gain.

I have had conversations with type 2 diabetics, who have had insulin added to their oral diabetes medicines. Some of them continue to gain weight, knowing the risks with every pound gained and becoming extremely frustrated. Unfortunately, some blame the weight gain solely on the insulin and not the food that they are eating. On the other hand, I have also met people who, despite being on insulin have been able to manage their weight very well.

I know several people who developed type I diabetes in childhood, who wear an insulin pump and have maintained their weight within a normal range. A good example of this is Manny, who had been on insulin for a very long time when we met. He achieved much in his career and lived a full life. He was also very disciplined about his food. His meals were portioned correctly. He never snacked. And, he walked a lot. He worked as a volunteer chair of a committee for a non-profit hospital well into his retirement, eventually passing away at the age of 80 from a heart attack. This was in the 1970s when 80 years of age was a decent life expectancy. For all the years on insulin, he remained slim throughout his life. The key was his consistent diet and exercise, which kept his blood sugar stable and insulin dose quite low. Admittedly, this type of lifestyle is very difficult to maintain. I have also met people who were on multiple oral diabetes medications plus insulin and came off insulin once they lost weight. Almost everyone with type 2 diabetes has a fear of adding insulin to their regimen. Because they believe that once they are on insulin, they can never come off insulin again. The key to getting the best benefit from insulin is for people with type 2 diabetes to manage their weight so that they can stay on the *lowest-effective dose* for as long as possible.

Reliance on Medications and Self-Deception

Essentially, there are two ways to lower blood glucose. The first is where the blood glucose is lowered, but the insulin resistance remains because of the type of medicine, or because the body weight is unchanged or increased. The second way is to lower blood sugar with medication, and at the same time lowering insulin resistance through weight management. People have more power than they realize to use medications to control their diabetes.

Then, there are some who eat without regard to their blood glucose levels, weight, overall health, or even the distress of their spouses, but they know just what to do before their doctor's visits. These patients never admit to their habits, but their laboratory results often give them away. Also, their spouses or family members would sometimes voice their concern about how they manipulated their blood glucose levels by being "good" a few weeks before the visit, just to get through the 15-minute visit and not get scolded too much. Clinics are busy places and it is impossible to have long talks about bad habits. And the patients know this, so, immediately after their doctor's visit, they go back to neglecting their diet until their next checkup in six months.

When they are first diagnosed with type 2 diabetes, people are not usually started on insulin, unless their blood glucose is extremely high, or it is an emergency. Typically, it is added when maximum doses of two or more oral diabetic drugs fail to control their blood sugar. As the blood sugar stabilizes with small doses of insulin, some people feel that their diabetes has been treated and feel comfortable about not watching their diet. At the next doctor's visits, their insulin dose may be increased as needed to maintain it at near normal levels, in other words, accommodating their lifestyle and eating habits. Insulin and diabetic medications do not cure diabetes, they simply lower blood glucose. It is the lowering of insulin resistance that truly helps to control the actual condition.

At a certain point, some people need larger doses and volumes of insulin. There are many types of insulin and one of the insulins that was felt to be a game changer was insulin glargine, a long-acting basal insulin, which was introduced about a decade ago. Today, there is a new formulation of insulin glargine which is three times more concentrated to accommodate those that need higher volumes. Some are resigned to using insulin long-term and feel it is the point of no return. Yet, there has been evidence that type 2 diabetes can be prevented to a certain degree with early and intensive diet and lifestyle changes.

Misunderstanding and Misuse of Medications

Many people, who have tried diets, exercise, meal plans, weight-loss groups, and supplements, tend to be very knowledgeable about the latest diets and weight loss plans available. However, they may still get frustrated from lack of progress, and turn to medications as a last resort.

One of my diabetic patients, Barbara, who was on an appetite suppressant, came into the office for a checkup. When she started on the appetite suppressants, she figured she could eat anything she wanted, and the medication would take care of it. She started eating ice cream every day and had gained seven pounds over four weeks. She proudly said she did take her diabetes medication in the evening, so the next morning her blood sugar would be near normal.

She had been instructed on portion control and carbs before starting the medication, but she had high expectations about the medication. Before getting on the scale, she warned the nurse, "I've been bad. My husband and I went out to eat a lot, and, I love ice cream. I'm addicted to it." They ate at restaurants several times a week. Prior to her visit, she had pizza three times during the week. After each restaurant meal, they would go to a frozen yogurt shop with a toppings bar, where you help yourself to different types of candy, chocolate and fruit. She had convinced herself that yogurt was healthy and the drug, metformin, would maintain her blood-sugar levels. No one was surprised when the scale showed she had gained weight. As you can see, the problem is relying on medications to do the work for you. Once she learned about the role of medications in her life, she corrected her eating habits and started to lose weight.

Another example is about three women who were seen separately in the clinic on the same day. All three were given the same instructions, the same type and dose of appetite suppressant, and information on diets and exercise. The following week, two had lost several pounds each; however, the third woman, Tammy, had gained two pounds. When asked about what she ate during the week, she said she had entertained a couple of times that week, drank a couple of glasses of wine every day, and had desserts throughout the week. The other two followed instructions, counted portions and calories, and limited carbs. Tammy relied on the appetite suppressants and ignored everything else.

The diabetic medication metformin had become a crutch for another patient, John, who worked and played hard. He had a stressful job as a business owner, and his favorite way to relax included going to happy hour, boating, fishing, and having cookouts with family and friends. This also meant lots of cold beer. Over the years, he gained a lot of weight and developed high blood pressure, high cholesterol, and diabetes. It got bad enough that he had a heart attack and ended up having a cardiac bypass.

John flat out refused to listen to his physician's advice and made sure everyone knew his lifestyle was going to remain exactly the same, and no one was going to take away his metformin. He said, how else could he keep drinking the amount of beer he had been drinking and still be alive? He knew that beer had a high glycemic index, which would interfere with his blood sugar control, yet he relied heavily on the medication and continued to experience poor health.

Elizabeth was a diabetic who struggled with her weight. She was already on two diabetic medications and her blood glucose was not under control. The staff had reviewed her diet many times to no avail. She couldn't exercise because her hips and knees hurt too much. I had broached the subject of adding insulin to her medications, but she hated injections. Meanwhile, she was beginning to get some numbness and tingling in her feet—early signs of diabetic peripheral neuropathy. Another medication was added to address these new symptoms, and I suggested insulin again. After a long discussion, she finally conceded, saying "Fine, I'll take the insulin. But you won't ever get me to give up my cheesecake. I have to have it every night or I can't sleep!" The comfort of eating cheesecake was more important than her overall health. She felt it was more important than controlling her blood glucose, which would have allowed her to have a better night's sleep than be kept awake by the tingling and numbness in her feet.

Finding Strength in Our Will Power

Whether it be diabetic medications or appetite suppressants, there are many highly effective medications available. As potent as these drugs are, in certain situations, we humans are stronger than the drugs. Some people can override the effect of insulin and some, the effect of appetite suppressants. In the chapter on motivation, we discussed the victim mentality and how some people trap themselves in a no-win situation. John and Elizabeth are examples of people who take medications so that they can maintain their lifestyle and have no interest at all in improving their disease. Barbara and Tammy honestly misunderstood how the medication should be used and once it was explained to them, they were able to get good results.

Approved Weight Loss Medications

The FDA has approved several medications to help with weight loss. Each medication has its own benefit and risk profile, as well as drug interactions. They all have maximum allowable doses and require monitoring with a medical provider. These medications are typically prescribed for individuals who are either overweight or obese.

Below is a list of FDA approved medications for weight loss.

- *Qsymia^{TM}*: A combination drug containing phentermine, an older appetite suppressant and topiramate. Topiramate can cause tingling and numbness in the feet.

- *Belviq^{TM}* (lorcaseran): This medication acts through the serotonin receptors. Although it acts through a different set of receptors than some antidepressant medications, there are precautions about using these drugs together.

- *Contrave^{TM}*: Combines bupropion and naltrexone. Bupropion is used for depression and to help people stop smoking. Naltrexone is an opioid antagonist used in drug addiction, and this medication may help in those with food addictions or cravings.

- *Saxenda^{TM}* or liraglutide: A medication used in diabetes and approved for weight loss, it works through the gastrointestinal tract to make you feel full earlier during a meal. On the other hand, it can cause some gastrointestinal upset.

- *Phentermine, Phendimetrazine* and *diethylpropion*: These medications belong to the stimulant class of drugs. They are typically used for short term weight loss. Side effects may include palpitations, dry mouth, and increased blood pressure.

- *Orlistat*: This medication affects the absorption of fat in the gastrointestinal tract. Therefore, those who use this medication should make sure to prevent deficiencies in fat soluble vitamins, A, D, E, and K. For some people, bloating and diarrhea may be side effects.

- *Vyvanse^{TM}* (lisdexamfetamine): A drug used for impulse control, it is typically prescribed for attention deficit hyperactive disorder (ADHD) in adults and children over the age of 6 years. It is approved by the FDA for the treatment of Binge Eating Disorder (BED) when it is associated with overweight and obesity.

- *Metformin*: A diabetes medication, it can cause gastrointestinal disturbances. It is useful when managing metabolic syndrome.

Commonly Used Drugs Associated with Weight Gain

There are medications that can cause weight gain. Corticosteroids can be life-saving in situations like asthma, meningitis, and lupus, because of the calming effect on inflammation. But, when corticosteroids are taken chronically, they cause side effects, including weight gain from fluid retention, and redistribution and deposition of fat around the face and the shoulders.

Insulin, sulfonylureas and thiazolidinediones are used to treat type 2 diabetes and can cause weight gain. On the other hand, drugs such as metformin and newer drugs, such as glucagon like peptide 1 (GLP-1) receptor agonists, and sodium glucose co-transporter (SGLT) 2 inhibitors, can help with weight loss.

Depression can be associated with weight gain, and some antidepressants can also contribute to weight gain, making matters worse. Older antidepressants such as amitriptyline, and nortriptyline, and paroxetine, a serotonergic drug can cause weight gain, whereas bupropion can help with weight loss.

Other drugs that are associated with weight gain include birth control pills and injections, antihypertensive drugs such as beta blockers, and some seizure medications. If there is any suspicion that a medication may be causing weight gain or preventing your efforts to lose weight, it should be discussed with your primary doctor to see if switching to a different drug might make a difference. That being said, not everyone responds to drugs in the same way. Some of my patients swear by a medication to help with osteoarthritis knee pain, and others say it is useless. Because, everyone responds differently, I believe both are correct. The best thing to do is to have an honest look at how you use your medications and have a discussion with your doctor. Some medical providers may tailor medications in different combinations based on their experience, which is considered off-label use.

When looking at medications, there is a difference between saying **A** *causes* **B**, and saying **A** is *associated* with **B**, even though some use the terms interchangeably. For example, a recent article described how ice cream sales were connected to shark bites. When ice cream sales went up, so did shark bites. This was considered a correlation. But, ice cream didn't cause the sharks to bite people. The article found an association between the two because there are more people on the beach during summer and more people eating ice cream.

So, for instance, when a statement says a certain medication for depression is associated with weight gain, we need to remember that depression by itself can be associated with weight gain in some people if they turn to food for comfort. Antidepressants do not treat the underlying cause of the depression, but they improve the mood of the individual, allowing them an opportunity to address the cause of their depression. If the individual stays on the medication, but the situation that caused the depression in the first place does not change, then it may seem that the medication is causing the weight gain. There are different medications to choose from and the best way to find out is by switching to a different medication for a while. Therapy and counseling is also a treatment method that is sometimes overlooked.

We are accustomed to having our doctors prescribe a medication to make something better or to make it go away. Very little effort is required on our part. Weight loss is different. Medical professionals were previously trained to treat conditions such as diabetes or hypertension promptly, but it was not until recently that obesity itself was recognized as a disease. Since then, we are urged to address overweight and obesity from day one. Even so, the reality is that medical professionals have very little control over how well an individual does once they leave the medical office. Make a goal to take back your life by controlling chronic medical conditions and to take as few medications as possible. And, by doing so, I hope you add years to your life and life to your years.

12. Cheers

"Not to get technical, but according to chemistry, alcohol is a solution."

Anonymous

"Once, during Prohibition, I was forced for days to live on nothing but food and water."

W.C. Fields

We all know that most alcoholic drinks have a lot of calories, especially sugary and fruity drinks, like the Mai Tai and Daiquiri. On the other hand, drinks like vodka and low carb beers are considered "diet friendly." Red wine also seems to have been elevated to "health food" status and I know people who drink red wine regularly for their health. I know many smart, ambitious, and successful people who can follow a diet perfectly, but draw a line at cutting back or eliminating alcohol, even temporarily, at the cost of undermining their own efforts. Some openly claim that they will compromise in other areas, except when it comes to alcohol. For others, the topic is simply not open for discussion.

Alcohol's "Empty" Calories Are Still Calories

Some of the calories in alcoholic drinks come from sugars and carbohydrates. The rest come from ethyl alcohol (all the calories in whiskey and vodka come from ethyl alcohol). Companies can label their drinks as "Zero Carbs," which is true, but the drink still has calories and are not truly empty. In terms of energy, ethyl alcohol produces 7 calories per gram[1], and carbohydrates provide 4 calories per gram. Fat has 9 calories per gram. The calories from ethyl alcohol provide energy through a different pathway and the byproduct of alcohol, acetaldehyde, is a toxin, which our body quickly eliminates. Energy from alcohol is produced through a complex pathway and has a surprising effect on digestion and metabolism.

Unlike most foods that are absorbed into the body through the small intestines, alcohol absorption begins in the stomach, where it competes with other nutrients involved in digestion, such as glucose, amino acids, and fat[2]. In other words, it "cuts through the line," interrupts the liver, and holds up the use of other nutrients and fat already in the body. Now, remember that fat is stored in the liver, subcutaneous, and visceral areas. For someone who is trying to lose fat, this means their body puts the brakes on the process each time alcohol is consumed. So, yes, we need to be concerned about the alcohol intake, whether we drink vodka, beer, or wine. But nutritional information about alcohol is not always readily available.

Where Are Those Nutrition Labels?

If you walk through the different sections of a supermarket, almost all packaged foods have a printed nutrition data chart with the contents listed. Today, many people are so focused on the quality of their food, and there are articles about how to choose the best of the best organic foods. There are many articles that tell us that some foods we ate growing up, are not worth eating or may be bad for us. Food information is everywhere, but when you get to the alcoholic beverages section in the grocery store, most of the bottles don't have any nutritional data[3]. Why are they exempted from listing this information?

The reason is simple. The Food and Drug Administration (FDA), the governing body that regulates food quality, does not regulate alcohol.

Alcohol is under the Alcohol and Tobacco Tax and Trade Bureau (TTB) that is part of the Department of Treasury. The FDA does very little with the TTB, a branch of government with little to no expertise on nutrition. It's just one of those things that make you go "Aha!" when you realize that alcohol is regulated under the Treasury that is also in charge of the Internal Revenue Service (IRS).

Alcohol is a controlled substance and heavily taxed. The alcoholic beverage market is a $354 billion industry, comprised of $211 billion in direct sales of beverages alone. It's safe to say that there is a lot of money involved, which means corporations aren't looking to curb America's appetite for booze any time soon.

What we see on bottles of beer or spirits is advertising. "Low Carb!" One light beer boasts "64 Calories." The TTB does not require nutrition labels on alcohol. It only requires the "Truthful and accurate factual statements about calorie and carbohydrate content in the labeling and advertising of alcohol" (TTB Ruling 2004-1). What they say is true and low carb means fewer than 8 grams of carbohydrates per 12 ounces of beer.

Just remember, these are not empty calories and ethyl alcohol throws a wrench in your digestive gears. But, then again, do people really want to know the nutritional content of their drinks? There has been an effort by some distillers and distributors to bring attention to some of the nutritional data. Across the industry, things are not going to change any time soon. So, who's complaining? This is one of those "blind spots" I'll talk about in the next chapter.

The Struggle with Changing Habits

We can't put our lives on hold when we go on a diet. That's why we need to understand our choices and create boundaries to lose weight. An example of making lifestyle choices to lose weight is Sophie, who is a young, outgoing, personable, and ambitious woman. When I met her, she was enrolled in a dual college degree program and working part time. She had plans to travel abroad with friends for a year after graduation. Meanwhile, juggling school and work had created a lot of stress, causing her to gain weight. She tried to exercise but couldn't shed those pounds. Eventually, she settled on a low carb diet.

Sophie was motivated by her research on low carb and ketogenic diets. She felt this would do the trick. She counted her portions and carbohydrates and followed her plan. After the first week, her results were very encouraging, even though she accepted that some of the weight loss was from water. She was in moderate ketosis and was getting used to a low carb regimen.

Beyond the first week though, her weight didn't budge. When she started her diet, there were some things she overlooked. She did not address how her social life was going to impact her weight loss efforts. She often went to happy hour after work. On the weekends, there were the beach parties and barbecues with friends. Even so, she was careful to avoid eating too many carbs. Her choice of drink up to this point had been beer, but she switched to vodka, because it had no carbs. The truth was, three vodkas several times a week wasn't doing her waistline any favors especially since she wasn't counting the calories from the drinks, because she considered them to be "empty" as in "zero."

I have another example that explains how a balanced diet is not enough to counter the effects of alcohol. Bethany had taken good care of her health all her life and was quite proud of it. She had never been obese, although with middle age, she had gained some extra weight and was now overweight. She ate what she considered to be a balanced diet. She took her vitamins, calcium and fish oil. When she read about the health benefits of red wine, she drank it regularly. At first, she drank just one glass a day, but when her husband passed, she started drinking a bit more, and then some more. She always kept a supply on hand to make sure she never ran out. She also stopped playing golf. It was something she and her husband had done together with other couples. Now, she felt like the fifth wheel. Bethany was quite surprised when, at the age of 66, she was diagnosed with diabetes.

From my experience, when dieters say they've had a bad week, I know that more often than not, alcohol is involved. The reasons vary from having company stay for an extended visit, or they went out of town to attend an event. I absolutely believe them when they say, "I tried really hard to be good about the food I ate." But, I do wonder about those who drink alcohol and how they manage the drinks. Remember our list of reasons why diets fail? The Triangle and Zones of Influence? These have a major effect on our ability to control our drinking, or to stop, even for a short time. When we drink, we lose our inhibitions which leads to eating more. It really does become a slippery slope.

At Restaurants and Bars

Some years ago, in the middle of the recession, people wanted to continue to eat out and still stay on a budget. Friends would go out and share appetizers and drinks, instead of ordering entrees. Many people didn't find it too hard to compromise this way and restaurants changed their menus to accommodate. We see more tapas and small plates on menus than before. And, honestly, the appetizers are probably more in line with what normal meal portions should be.

In a Tampa Bay Times article, Greg Baker, owner and chef of the restaurant Fodder and Shine, was quoted, "People claim they want healthier, but they really want fat, rich and decadent. That said, folks will still pony up big bucks in one area—booze. Even as diners demand lower priced dishes, they will splurge on a mojito. The menu may be burgers, but that pint of craft beer is still going to be $5."

Meeting your friends for happy hour on Fridays, or several times a week like Sophie did, can undermine all of your efforts during the week. Appetizers and drinks are becoming more decadent—more fun—unless you are trying to lose weight. A martini is gin and vermouth. Today, there are so many different types of martinis, including crowd favorites like the chocolate martini and cosmopolitan. The chocolate martini has more than 425 calories. That's more than three glasses of wine worth of calories.

All Things in Moderation

Moderate alcohol consumption is defined as one drink per day for women and two drinks per day for men[4]. Among the small pockets of communities where people live to be age 100 and over, there is no indication that they live to be centenarians because they are abstinent. For dieters, the simplest way to manage alcohol calories, since there is no nutrition label to go by, is to calculate the total calories per drink (shown below) in the daily calories consumed. It is better if you still limit your daily net carb intake.

The only piece of information hard liquor, such as whiskey, scotch, and vodka, is required to show is percent proof. Beer and wine are not required to have anything on their label if their percentage of alcohol is at or below a certain threshold. The story behind the term *proof* goes back to the 18th century in the United Kingdom. If a pellet of gunpowder soaked in alcohol could be lit on fire, it was "above proof" and had enough alcohol in it to not be considered watered down[4]. Today, the definition of proof is simply multiplying the alcohol content by 2. For example, 40% alcohol equals 80 proof.

It is as though the bottles are mocking us, saying "That's it! Take it or leave it." The general, unwritten message seems to be, if you are old enough to drink alcohol, you must be old enough to disregard the lack of nutritional data. Besides, nobody drinks alcohol as a main part of their diet, or do they? You may be out to dinner with friends, and choose to forego the wine, because of all those calories from sugar. Instead, you get a whiskey and diet cola. Now, you're thinking you can have a few bites of dessert, later. Not that you can't, but don't forget to add the calories from your drink to your total intake for the day.

A standard drink contains about 14 grams of alcohol. That's almost 100 calories! Now, think about that no carb drink. It may not have any calories associated with carbs, but it does have 100 calories of alcohol. Below is a table of calories for alcoholic drinks[5], and a link for calculating total alcoholic calories per week[6].

Alcoholic Beverage Calorie Chart

BEVERAGE	SERVING SIZE	CALORIES
Beer		
Beer (light)	12 oz.	103
Beer (regular)	12 oz.	153
Beer (craft beers)	12 oz.	170 to 420
Distilled Alcohol		
Gin (80 proof)	1.5 oz.	97
Gin (94 proof)	1.5 oz.	116
Rum (80 proof)	1.5 oz.	197
Rum (94 proof)	1.5 oz.	116
Vodka (80 proof)	1.5 oz.	97
Vodka (94 proof)	1.5 oz.	116
Whiskey (80 proof)	1.5 oz.	97
Whiskey (94 proof)	1.5 oz.	116
Liqueurs		
Coffee liqueur	1.5 oz.	160
Coffee liqueur with cream	1.5 oz.	154
Crème de menthe	1.5 oz.	186
Mixed Drinks		
Bloody Mary	5 oz.	120
Chocolate martini	6.5 oz.	438
Cosmopolitan	4 oz.	200
Daiquiri	6 oz.	337

Highball	8 oz.	110
Hot buttered rum	8 oz.	292
Mai Tai	6 oz.	350
Margarita	8 oz.	280
Mimosa	4 oz.	75
Mint Julep	4.5 oz.	165
Mojito	8 oz.	214
Pina colada	4.5 oz.	245
Rum and Coke	8 oz.	185
Rum and Diet Coke	8 oz.	100
Tequila sunrise	6.8 oz.	232
Vodka and tonic	8 oz.	200
Whiskey sour	6 oz.	289
White Russian	8oz.	568

Wine

White table wine	5 oz.	121
Gewurztraminer	5 oz.	119
Muscat	5 oz.	123
Riesling	5 oz.	118
Chenin Blanc	5 oz.	118
Chardonnay	5 oz.	123
Sauvignon Blanc	5 oz.	119
Fume Blanc	5 oz.	121
Pinot Grigio	5 oz.	122
Dry dessert wine	3.5 oz.	157
Red table wine	5 oz.	125
Petite Syrah	5 oz.	125

Merlot	5 oz.	122
Cabernet Sauvignon	5 oz.	122
Red Zinfandel	5 oz.	129
Burgundy	5 oz.	127
Pinot Noir	5 oz.	121
Claret	5 oz.	122
Syrah	5 oz.	122
Red dessert wine	3.5 oz.	165

Our Love Affair with Booze

The Prohibition Era proved our love affair with alcohol. We have it during celebrations, parties, or simply watching TV. Each year, the alcohol beverage industry finds new and inventive ways to increase their profits. Ads for alcohol bombard us everywhere, and for some people these ads are a little too convincing. College students are affected by binge drinking and some may continue these habits after college. And, chronic alcohol abuse leads to many diseases, especially of the liver (cirrhosis) and the heart (cardiomyopathy). Being aware of the amount of alcohol you drink is very important to your overall health and well-being.

Like food, alcohol is inert, and ultimately, we decide to consume it, which determines our success or failure in managing our weight. Those who take calories from alcohol into account will always have an advantage over those who overlook it. The lure of alcohol is obvious to restauranteurs, alcoholic beverage manufacturers and to TTB. Revenue from alcohol sales will never suffer in good times or bad.

As intelligent consumers, we can educate ourselves to be aware of the impact of alcohol on our weight and on our health. Just because the regulatory bodies don't count the calories on the labels, it doesn't mean that we should also fail to count them, because our bodies certainly are counting. Managing our weight does not mean giving up alcohol completely, but moderating its intake and when there is some immediate need to lose weight, foregoing alcohol temporarily. will reap better rewards.

13. Blind Spots

"It is useless to attempt to reason a man out of a thing he was never reasoned into."

Jonathan Swift, Irish writer and satirist

"Real knowledge is to know the extent of one's ignorance."

Confucius (Chinese philosopher, 500 B.C.)

The chapter on Zones of Influence discussed invisible boundaries that need to be established when interacting with people close to us, such as family members, coworkers, and friends. This chapter focuses on how we may not always see things as they are, when dealing with our environment. A good example of this phenomenon occurred in 2015, when a picture went viral on the internet, simply asking viewers what the color of a dress was. Some people said it was blue and black. Others swore that it was white and gold. The dress was actually blue and black, but when viewed under a different level of light or a different angle, it somehow looked white and gold. If simply changing the light had millions of people's opinion divided, think about all that we see or hear and process on a daily basis. Sometimes, when we realize our interpretations are off the mark, we can quickly correct ourselves. Other times, the shaping of our views and our opinions are the product of repeated subtle social cues, which cause "blind spots" in our perception. Anais Nin said, "We don't see things as they are, we see them as we are."

Even when we have 20/20 vision, we see the world around us with a filtered lens that affects our perceptions. Sometimes, we encounter people who come across as having their filters slightly askew; their words and actions may speak more about themselves than the target or subject of their words. How we interact with them also says something about who we are, and our own filters, or blind spots. These interactions can happen in public, or during a more private moment between two people, and we consciously or unconsciously turn a "blind eye". Sometimes, we do it for the sake of civility, and at other times, it is because we are oblivious to our own shortcomings.

Going through life and interacting with others, we live within the boundaries of social norms such as politeness, courtesy and consideration. There are too many people living in the world, and in the absence of these unspoken rules, we would destroy each other very quickly. Since "an eye for an eye would make the world blind," we develop "blind spots" to help us live in some level of harmony. Blind spots can be an adaptive measure for us to maneuver through and interact with our environment, but sometimes they can cause us to be insensitive, and at other times even cause us to be gullible. As you read this chapter, you will recognize different blind spots including those used by the marketing and advertising industry.

What You Don't Know May Hurt You: Becoming Self-Aware

A study in 2008[1] shows how we are not very good at guessing whether our weight falls in the normal, overweight, or obese category. Among the study volunteers, only 22.2% of obese women and 6.7% of obese men correctly classified themselves as obese. They thought they had to weigh quite a bit more to be considered obese. On the other hand, men and women who were in the normal weight range thought they didn't have to put on too much weight to be considered obese. When they gave the weight at which they thought they would be obese, researchers noted that the average BMI was only 28.9, which is the overweight category. But, when women who were obese gave the researchers the weight at which they thought they would be obese, it matched up with a BMI of 38.2, which is class 2 obesity.

Why does this matter? The authors noted that people who were overweight or obese could possibly disregard any public health messages about obesity related conditions, thinking it would not apply to them because they didn't think they were as heavy as they really were. They may also ignore any advice from health professionals about losing weight.

This misperception has also been found to be true among teenagers[2, 3]. A study in the American Journal of Preventive Medicine reported results from how teens thought about their weight over two different periods. The first group included teenagers from 1988 – 1994. A second, separate group of teenagers were surveyed about ten years later, from 2007 – 2012. When we look at these time frames, we know that obesity rates throughout the world had increased by the second survey. Yet, fewer obese and overweight teens in the second survey thought that they were overweight or obese. Many thought they were just about the right weight.

Although this may seem surprising, there is probably a good reason. To put things in perspective, I believe that it is fair to assume that the teenagers in both studies formed their perceptions of their own weight from their families and their environments, years before they became teenagers. Also, adult obesity rates were a lot lower in the first study period, and modern conveniences were not as easily accessible. We could generally assume that the parents of the teens in the earlier study were more likely to be of normal weight than the parents of the teens in the later study. If a child belonged to a family where both parents are carrying some extra pounds, and they share the same meals, over the years, the child would simply adopt similar lifestyles and habits. If you, your parents, and your siblings look similar, then that becomes perfectly normal to you. Every child gets their bearings and reference points from their core families, and their role models are the parents or guardians. When their perceptions have been skewed from an early age, and if no one corrects them, they are set on a different course, possibly for the rest of their lives.

The problem with such misperceptions is that the added weight causes health problems as we grow older. A recent study looked at female nurses and male health professionals from the time they were young adults to age 55[4]. The researchers found that, among both groups, those who became overweight or obese had more health problems such as type 2 diabetes, high blood pressure, heart disease, cataracts, and severe arthritis. The following is an example of how such misperceptions play out at an individual level.

Linda and Dean had a successful business, which involved driving to different customer businesses throughout the state to install machine parts. They kept their overhead low by doing everything themselves. This meant accepting and making orders, driving, installing the parts during the day and keeping the accounts straight at night. Because of this, they were always eating on the run, or eating take out. Their weights had increased significantly, but they decided that they were still just a bit overweight. When their blood pressures and cholesterol levels started to increase, their primary care doctor advised them to lose weight. Dean thought this was not a bad idea, but Linda didn't think there was a problem with her weight and she just needed to watch what she ate.

Nevertheless, she agreed to go with Dean to see the nutritionist. After introductions, Linda and Dean were asked to step onto the scales to calculate their weight, BMI, fat percent, and lean mass. The nutritionist explained that this would be their baseline and she would be developing individual plans for them. Linda became very upset and agitated. She told the nutritionist she did not know her weight, didn't want to know her weight, and refused to step on the scale. She said she didn't have a weight problem and had come only as a favor to her doctor. Dean shrugged and said it was no big deal, and stepped on the scale, while Linda peeked at the number on the scale and giggled. Throughout the visit, Linda teased Dean about his weight, made sarcastic remarks to the nutritionist, and flat out told her she refused to use a journal, count calories, or to allow anyone to weigh her. The nutritionist did not argue, and only encouraged them to focus on eating healthier. Dean absorbed all the information and followed instructions, and the results showed. Linda did not return. This was until one day, Linda started having chest pains at work. Startled, she checked in at the emergency room and realized she was having a heart attack. She ended up with a stent, and this became the turning point for her lifestyle change.

This next example is about a morbidly obese young teen, who struggled to lose weight. His father proudly revealed that he knew all about losing weight. He had read all the latest articles, and basically gave me a great lecture on weight loss. Indeed, he had a wealth of knowledge. He had a plan for the two of them to go to the gym and go on a high-protein diet. He was obviously very eager to show his son the ropes. As I wished them luck, I noted that throughout the conversation, the son mostly avoided eye contact with me. Later, I happened to talk to his mother who told me that her son had been working hard on his own and making some progress, but none of his efforts had been acknowledged by the father. Evidently, the father felt that the son was an embarrassment to him and would comment about the son being an underachiever. He would regularly and loudly compare his son to his friends' children and how he was being made to look bad. About a year later, I learned that the young man was unable to lose any weight and had lap band surgery. I think that the father was so focused on himself and his own agenda that he failed to recognize any efforts made by his son. It probably made his son invisible, in the sense that his feelings, as well as his efforts, were ignored. No one wants to live as an invisible, excluded being, and it causes major damage to our self-esteem when we are invisible to the most important figure in our lives.

Acceptance, Fat shaming, and Accommodation

Another blind spot comes in the form of acceptance and accommodation. Acceptance is when people intentionally make excuses for morbid obesity. They say it is ok to carry as many excess pounds as we want regardless of our health and wellbeing and do nothing about it. This is wrong, but people prefer not to address it, because it is viewed as being insensitive. We need to think about this seriously. If we say that morbid adult obesity is okay, then the message to children is that childhood obesity and adult obesity are okay. Then, what will the health of these children be like as they grow older and is there no limit to excess weight at all?

On the other hand, weight is a very personal and private matter and "fat shaming" people into losing weight is wrong. Fat shamers are looking for one thing only, and that is a reaction to their cruel comments. They get satisfaction from seeing strong emotions, such as shock, disbelief, hurt, humiliation, and embarrassment. This is a major character flaw that fat shamers have and the worst part of it is that they are completely unaware of it. If people don't react to them with the expected emotions, their comments and actions are blunted. We all know people who carry extra weight who we regard highly. We should be judged for our character and personality, not our weight.

Compassion and support are different than blind acceptance, but it is also important to not send the wrong message to the next generation. We need to think about the legacy that we leave to our children. How many of us wish for our children to develop diabetes or fatty liver disease at a young age? Yet, this is happening. In a recent conversation with a bariatric surgery specialist, she lamented how she was seeing younger patients coming in for surgery. This is a tragedy. We need to give our children a chance at a healthy life.

Accommodation is a more complex matter. The health care system has also contributed to it. No matter how much it becomes accepted, obesity has serious health effects. Traditionally, the medical profession was trained to treat chronic medical conditions with medications. We were not taught in school how to deal with obesity until more recently. In a way, we had our blinders on and that is also a form of accommodation. The reality for health professionals is that we must work within a limited time frame of a clinic visit. Other legitimate medical problems must be addressed, and the patient also has their own priorities. And then, let's face it. Not everyone is receptive to our advice. This means that matters related to obesity go unaddressed. In addition, medical care is dictated by the health insurance industry, which would pay for treatment of chronic diseases rather than prevention. In the past, there were times when I felt as though I was simply helping the patient keep their chronic disease condition by not having the capability to address their weight problem. In other words, I felt that I was accommodating their illness and not addressing the root cause.

Today, there is more awareness of diseases related to obesity. Public health agencies suggest a more pro-active management of obesity, giving it equal importance as other chronic diseases. This makes more sense than prescribing increasingly higher doses of medications to treat cardiovascular disease or diabetes. Adding more medications as people continue to gain weight may control the laboratory data and make people feel better, but unless it is accompanied by weight management, it will not improve their overall health and quality of life.

Some diseases related to obesity, such as cancer, can affect an entire family. As mentioned in an earlier chapter, breast cancer is one of the cancers associated with obesity[5]. While there are genetic factors that can lead to breast cancer, obesity remains one of the modifiable risks among those without a genetic risk. Risk factors that have been associated with cancer include alcohol, low physical activity and obesity. According to the American Cancer Society[6], excess weight is associated with one out of five deaths from cancer.

Sheila is an example of someone who needed to modify her lifestyle, but decided not to, and chose to take medications for her health-related problems. She had worked hard her entire life, but her job and lifestyle had always been sedentary. She took medications for her diabetes and to control her high cholesterol and blood pressure. When she was diagnosed with breast cancer, she had been morbidly obese for years and never tried to diet or exercise. She had a mastectomy to remove both breasts and the lymph nodes in her armpits. Her recovery was difficult and painful. She also had breast reconstruction, which became infected. In addition, the medications she took for the cancer caused extreme nausea and vomiting. It was difficult to take care of herself and work, and she ultimately lost her job.

Sheila needed help to do things she had always done on her own. Little things, like brushing her hair and dressing herself became painful because of the scarring, pain and swelling in her arms. She was forced to move in with her daughter, who had two small children. The stress of taking care of her mother and two young children affected her daughter to the point where she would yell at her kids for insignificant things. Sheila had become a burden for her daughter, something no parent would wish for their children.

Gordon's friends and family affectionately referred to him as "big Gordon." He was 6 feet 3 inches tall and weighed 360 pounds. His BMI was 45, or morbidly obese. For many years, he was a tow truck driver and an avid motorcyclist. He rarely exercised and ate whatever he wanted. He would become upset if any health care provider brought up his weight. He had gone through several physicians and told funny stories to his friends and family about how he fired one idiot. doctor after another.

One early morning on a winding mountain road, a deer suddenly ran out in front of him and his bike. When he hit the deer, his lower body was thrown violently against the handle bars. The impact shattered his pelvis and the transmitted force broke his lower spine, one leg, and his knee. When he came to, he felt fortunate to be alive, while friends and family rallied around.

Over the next year, he underwent multiple surgeries and hours of rehabilitation. The surgeon's operative notes mentioned the difficulty of the surgeries, because of the amount of fat. Fortunately, for Gordon, the operations were successful. However, Gordon's recovery and continued rehabilitation were not smooth. Learning to walk again was an extremely painful process. His pelvis and knees struggled to support his weight. Eventually, he walked again with the help of a cane, but continued to live with chronic pain. He could no longer work at his job. He became irritable and mean to his wife, who helped take care of him. He never understood why they couldn't make him whole again. In the end, Gordon's choices affected the people he loved.

Media and Body Image

We frequently see articles on the internet or in popular magazines that tempt you to click on headlines, such as "See how amazing these celebrities look after losing 100 pounds." You never see a headline inviting you to look at an amazing picture of someone after they gained 100 pounds. Why is this? Directly and indirectly, the information highway trains our minds to accept certain ideals of body images. All this while we are urged to accept morbid obesity. There needs to be more celebration of health than looks, but there aren't. They say a picture is worth a thousand words, and pictures and images are used so much by advertisers to send quick, high-impact messages to us, but it doesn't mean that they always have a positive value.

Advertising is meant to convince people to buy something, sometimes using people's insecurities and fears to do it. These tactics focus a large amount of money on sexually objectified images of young women in advertisements, some on billboards, wearing lingerie or string bikinis. These may be the ideal image for advertisers, but it is not a healthy representation of body types. Some magazines and media outlets are trying to break the mold but are slow to change their ways. This is a blind spot because some women feel pressured to be that thin, and in extreme cases, this type of advertising may cause young women to have eating disorders.

Television, magazines, and social media are the biggest contributors to our overall body image and how we compare ourselves with others. Our impressions about our body are formed every day when we look in the mirror. A positive body image comes from recognizing our physical shape and size, consisting of a healthy weight and curves.

We experience a serious disconnect with our body image when we want to look like someone, such as a model, but are nearly a foot shorter and have a stouter bone structure, larger breasts, or thick muscles. The negative perceptions affect our behavior and may keep us from feeling secure about ourselves. Negative body image is a serious problem for some young girls and women, leading to unhealthy lifestyles.

One of the ways to counteract this product of the media is to understand what your body type is and to be secure in the fact that it's who you are, and you are beautiful. Currently, there are three main categories for body types[7]:

Ectomorph – a slender frame, narrow shoulders, flat chest, lean muscles and high metabolism.
Mesomorph – medium sized bone structure, athletic, rectangular body shape, easily gains muscle.
Endomorph – large bone structure, generally short, stocky, and round physique with little muscle definition, and slow metabolism.

These are general categories, and everyone shares qualities among the three, rarely fitting the description of one category. Knowing which one you fit into may help you dismiss those obtrusive billboards on your way home from work.

Here is a good example from clothing stores. Some stores have resized their clothing, labeling a dress size 1, when in fact it is a 6. This artificial resizing of clothing is an apparent attempt to make people more comfortable purchasing clothes. At the same time, mannequins around the world have undergone a metamorphosis. Female mannequins used to be 5 feet 10 inches with a 26-inch waist. Today, they are six feet tall and have a 24-inch waist. An article stated that if these female mannequins were real humans, they would be so undernourished that they would not menstruate.

Among our five senses, sight, hearing, smell, touch and taste, our vision and hearing have the longest range, and therefore, we tend to process this sensory input to guide us before using the other senses, which are considered the "contact senses." Therefore, first impressions from advertising and television can make a great impact on our perceptions and how we make judgements, whether they turn out to be true or not. It's important to differentiate what the internet and media would suggest to us as positive role models and switch our reference point to real and valid sources.

We would not think of relying on a glossy home magazine's pictures to purchase a home. When selling a house, realtors and sellers know the importance of curb appeal. Yet, it's the cracked foundation, leaky roof, broken plumbing, and faulty electrical wiring that will pose major problems for the undiscerning homebuyer. We hire an inspector to go through the house to find what needs to be fixed, so we can make an informed decision. The same can be said about physicians and health professionals. When they perform a physical exam, order labs, mammograms, and x-rays, they are doing a clinical inspection. We should take our physical health cues from our health professionals to determine our ideal weight and health and not the internet, television, or magazines. When your primary care professional tells you that you are within a normal weight range, and your labs came back good, it should give you the validation you need.

Gathering a Realistic Picture of Ourselves and Those around Us

A health decision model known as the *Stages of Change* allows health professionals to determine where a patient's frame of mind is in making a lifestyle change. Based on the model, we assess whether someone is in one of the following stages:

- **Precontemplation** – Individuals unwilling or unable to think about changing their behavior.
- **Contemplation** – Individuals willing to consider the possibility of a problem.
- **Commitment to Action** – The decision to act has been made and individuals are following a course of action.

People move through these stages at their own pace. Far too many remain in the precontemplation phase and do not progress to action, like Sheila and Gordon, who disregarded warnings from their health care providers about losing weight. They went so far as to deny their failing health as anything but a natural course of events. About ten years ago, I saw a viral email that summed this topic of blind spots. It stated the following:

Watch your thoughts for they become words; watch your words for they become actions; watch your actions for they become your

habits; and, watch your habits, for they become your destiny. –
Frank Outlaw

Until we see marketing ploys for what they are, we will continue to accept them as valid points of reference. We will continue to have an obesity epidemic and miserable people of normal weight. We must align with our medical professionals and their knowledge, as well as be our own healthy lifestyle advocate. We can empower ourselves to ignore those people around us that are false experts and become more aware of our bodies and minds, how we think, and what "healthy" means to us. We have seen how the larger environment outside of our families can manipulate our perception, or blindsides us from time to time, but this also happens within families.

14. Modern Family Dynamics

"To love and to be loved is to feel the sun from both sides."

David Viscott

Parents influence their children's weight. Scientific research over the past three decades has confirmed this. Children mimic their parents' eating habits starting at a young age when they have no control over their food choices, and this is when eating habits begin to form.

As a parent, I understand the challenges of feeding my family. If we look at our modern lifestyle, we are in a constant battle against time: time to make the right choices and time to prepare healthy options. Fast food restaurants and pre-made meals, full of preservatives and fat, are there for us to save time. And, let's face it, many adults who face the challenges of being overweight and or obese grew up in households with similar lifestyles and food habits that became their norm.

The best part of being a parent is being blessed with having another person to love unconditionally. Making them happy makes us happy. We can feel it when they are sad or stressed. And, when they are hungry, we can easily remedy it with a snack from the cupboard. No wonder snack foods are now a multi-billion-dollar industry. It uses food sciences to know what tastes and looks best, so people will buy their product. Unfortunately, those snacks are loaded with sugar and fat, a compact source of calories.

As busy parents, we want to keep our children comfortable, and many of us are guilty of sometimes giving them a bag of chips to "hold them over until dinner," but this type of love may cause harm over time. In extreme cases, children may become morbidly obese. There is also such a thing as too much of a good thing, especially when it comes to food. Reflecting on previous chapters, we know how portion sizes are important, even when we eat those so-called superfoods, claiming to make us slim and healthy. Sure, they have a great list of nutritious ingredients, but eating too much has the opposite effect. The same could be said of our relationships with our children and our spouses. I think this concept is best served through some poignant examples I've come across during my years as a physician.

The Modern Mother

Time is a precious commodity in Diana's household. She is a full-time working mom with two children. Her husband commutes over a hundred miles round-trip, every day, to work in a high pressure managerial job. By the time they all sit down for dinner, it's after eight. That's eight hours between lunch and dinner, while it's only three to four hours between breakfast and lunch. Of course, the kids are hungry, so she gives them a late afternoon snack to hold them over until their dad gets home. She feels the pressure to make sure the kids don't go hungry. There are always bags of cookies and chips in the cupboard and juice in the fridge. On nights when she is pressed for time, she takes shortcuts for dinner, like Chinese take-out or stopping at a fast food restaurant.

Diana's eight-year old daughter, Charlotte, is overweight. She doesn't like sports, dance, or other physical activities. She would rather do coloring, read, or draw. And she is not a picky eater. Diana's four-year old son, Josh, is different from his sister, because he doesn't like to eat. He picks at his food and goes back to his activities after a few bites. He is also very active and loves sports. Diana worries about his weight, as much as she worries about Charlotte's, but for the opposite reason. She tries to tempt Josh to eat more, buying cookies, chips, pop tarts, anything to get him to eat. Diana is in a situation where she feels she must treat the two children very differently. Over time, except for Josh, their weights have crept up, and now Diana's husband is having health problems. Blood pressure and cholesterol medicines are now part of his daily life. And yet, Diana still feels obligated to participate in fund-raising activities such as bake-sales and other school and social activities surrounding the children and her family with food.

The Sandwich Generation

Recently, I met with a family friend to catch up on the latest events in her life. She is a highly educated health professional and a dedicated daughter. An important goal in her life was to help her parents when they became too old to care for themselves. At this point, she was a successful nursing professional and attending medical school. Despite many attempts to lose weight, she had slowly and steadily gained weight. She admitted that, she was frustrated with her continued weight gain.

She said, "My problem is carbs. I can't seem to resist them. My dad keeps telling me to lose weight. He even offered to buy me one of those programs that ship food to your house. He told me it doesn't matter how much it costs, just do it. He is literally begging me to lose weight. He is so funny. He worries so much about me."

I replied, "I don't think your dad is being funny. Do you think he is worried about you, or worried for himself and your mother because of you? Have you ever looked at it that way? That one day, you might be in poorer health than they are, and that in their old age, they might be taking care of you, because you had a heart attack, diabetes, cancer, or stroke?"

She looked stunned and paused to process what I had just asked. Then, she said, "I never thought about that."

This is a very close-knit family. Yet, in pursuing the best career opportunities to support the family, the parents had ended up living in two different countries, while the daughters went to college and pursued their careers in other countries. The parents had gone to great lengths to make sure that their daughters had stability while they were pursuing their college degrees. After their daughters became more established, the parents remained global nomads, seeing each other a few times a year while trying to save for retirement, so they could finally live together.

My friend continued, "Now that I think about it, my dad was out of work for a few years before he found his present job. At that time, he started working out every day while he was looking for a job. Some people thought he was going to the gym because he was just bored. But, I realize now that he was trying to keep himself in the best physical shape possible, so that he wouldn't get ill and become a burden to my mom. We were kids back then, but I remember him being so worried for our health. I had assumed that he just worked out because he wanted to look good."

It is one thing to say you love someone, but if your actions place them in a vulnerable position, the words are hollow and lack meaning. People on the receiving end may feel that even though they are hearing the words, something is missing, and they lack sincerity. On the other hand, you can do something out of love without saying a word and the other party may not appreciate it and may not even know about it. It is only when we reflect on actual behaviors that we can truly appreciate our families and friends and realize we have taken them for granted.

My friend had everything she needed. She had a great job, bright career prospects, a nice house, a luxury car, and free access to a top-of-the-line gym through her job. She just needed to stop seeing her father as the funny guy who kept harping on about her weight for no reason. She had to understand the precarious position he was in and stop taking him for granted. He wanted to retire, but in today's economy, many people have had to put off retirement because of the fear of not having enough money for themselves, let alone having to worry about the health of the next generation. One of the greatest gifts that any of us can give to those we love, is our good health.

For many of us who are in the age group that is often called the sandwich generation, the generation still taking care of their children and parents, the challenges seem endless. Our aging parents have needs that demand our time and energy, while our children, who are becoming young adults, struggle to stand on their feet. Some of us will never see retirement. The one thing that every one of us can give our families is the peace of mind that comes from them not having to worry about our health. The gift of good health is much better than Mother's Day brunch, or presents on Father's Day, or even an anniversary dinner. A long time ago, a respected relative said, "I will not be a burden to you. I plan to carry my old bones to my grave." Now, at 93, she has outlived many of her peers and is still in remarkably good health. *Words may be sweet, but actions speak louder.*

Being Conscious and Cautious

Kids are often caught between a rock and a hard place. They are told they shouldn't eat as much as they can, and that they should eat healthy foods. Yet, the same parent or teacher demonstrates the opposite behavior. It's like saying, "You'd better behave," then *wink-wink* at them, dismissing what you said.

My friends William and Mala are successful business owners, and they have two children: Jared is 12, and Grace is 9. The family leads busy lives and socializes frequently. Over time, William and Jared have gained a substantial amount of weight. One night, our families went to a popular restaurant that offered meals on a Hibachi grill. As the smell of cooking meat filled the room, Jared started helping himself. His dad admonished him, as he had numerous times, about eating too much and putting on too much weight. But, even as he said this, he was placing food on Jared's plate. At the end of the meal, William said to Jared, "That's it. You are coming with me for a walk tonight to burn off all that food." A ridiculous statement, when you really think about it, because they would need to walk for a very long time to burn those calories. Jared, I noticed, simply focused on his plate and seemed to tune his dad out, because he had probably heard it before.

No parent teaches bad food habits to their children on purpose. Parents want to give their children the best childhood they can provide, but teaching our children to be disciplined and wanting to reward them can send conflicting messages. Jared could have been taught about portions at home, instead of being criticized at the restaurant. Being embarrassed like this in public sets up the child for a negative self-image as they grow older.

Children Mimic Their Parents' Actions

According to child development experts, when children are around eight years old, about third grade, they transition from learning to read to reading to learn. This is a critical time in their development, because they are learning about autonomy, and forming independent views of their world. Children take their knowledge from their parents and teachers, then apply it to their daily lives. In class, they read and learn. At home, they play and do chores.

Experts also believe that this is one of the most important times in a child's life for parents to act as a role model. Parental guidance and engagement is important for children to make sound, healthy decisions. This becomes even more crucial in their teenage years, when peer relationships become a stronger influence while they must still rely on the strength and consistency of their family.

Healthy eating is also a modeled habit, and Jared and William's story has some scientific basis to it. Two research studies[1] looked at the correlation between obese children and obese parents. Both found that if the father was obese, it more than doubled the risk of the child being obese. The risk was tripled if the mother was obese. On the other hand, the children were not at risk of being obese when the parents were of normal weight. Also, researchers found[2] that when parents lost weight, their children also lost weight. Healthy habits begin in the home, which may seem obvious or make sense, but many times parents lose sight of that in our modern lifestyles.

The Right Kind of Support: Nicky

Childhood obesity is the result of complex and challenging family dynamics, economic and environmental situations, parents' lack of understanding nutrition, and their ability to manage weight. Most of the time, it's not that the parents do not care, rather, it's because they care too much. Loving and caring are like the sun. The warmth of the sun is pleasant and comfortable; yet, as the sun rises higher in the sky and gets hotter, UV factor increases along with the risk of getting sunburn. The same is true for children who suffer the consequences of their parent's adoration. While parents try to juggle the different needs of their children and one or more child becomes obese, they desperately search for answers. During this search, children may suffer from damage to their self-esteem.

When I met Nicky, I was told that the school and her parents were concerned about her weight and she was depressed. I later learned that the school had asked for a meeting with her parents about Nicky's cutting. Nicky didn't feel good about her weight or herself. Her parents fought about her eating too much, which deeply hurt her feelings. She didn't know what to do, and felt helpless, so she started cutting herself.

Cutting and other forms of self-harm are more common than one would think. It is estimated that about a quarter of adolescent girls actively cut themselves with fingernails, pen caps, or things that are much sharper[3]. It serves as a distraction from emotional pain. Cutting is a symptom of something much more serious happening to them and requires immediate attention. It's a signal for parents, family members, and teachers to intervene.

Nicky's dad worked extremely hard to provide for the family, and she was the apple of his eye. The mother was the homemaker, and Nicky had a younger sister, who was twelve. On the day of the meeting with the school administrators, her mother went, because her father couldn't get off from work. Her mother doesn't speak English very well and couldn't understand much of the discussion. At the end of the meeting, they were referred to a psychiatrist, who put Nicky on medication.

The family lived in another state and were brought to my home by a mutual friend. During the visit, her father explained that they were desperate to do something about Nicky's weight. At this point, they were contemplating gastric sleeve surgery and they wanted my opinion. Nicky's father invited her to ask me any questions about weight loss and she responded, "What questions?" Not unusual for a shy teenager receiving more attention than she wanted about a deeply personal matter. She was there physically, but not yet engaged in the discussion we were having.

At one point, her father exclaimed, "She just eats so much!" I turned to Nicky and asked if she wanted the surgery. She smiled, and said, "Sure." As we continued to talk, I discovered that she had periodically tried some diets with short term limited success. She would do well for a week and then give up. So, I asked, "If you had a choice between diet and exercise or surgery, which would you choose?" She said, "There is no choice," then corrected herself, "It doesn't matter."

For any diet to work, she needed to stay on it for more than one week. And unless she changed her eating habits, the chances of her being able to keep the weight off in the long term was questionable. Even more important, the entire family had to make changes in their diet or else Nicky was doomed to fail.

As bariatric surgery was an elective surgery, I asked if she would consider giving herself a few months to consistently diet and exercise before moving forward with the surgery, knowing this would give her a better chance of maintaining her weight loss afterwards. She agreed and became engaged in the conversation. She was quite knowledgeable about basic nutrition facts and she liked to read. I was impressed by Nicky's knowledge about different diets, and I pointed out to her that she already knew many things. She was pretty, intelligent, and hopefully getting motivated to lose weight.

I asked them to describe their typical days and meals. They had stopped buying regular soda, only to replace it with fruit juices. They drank whole milk. They also had an endless supply of chips and cookies.

As we talked, the younger daughter had put her head down in her mother's lap, tuning everyone out. Nicky's mother defended her grocery choices, and said, "Well, I still have to think about her," while looking at her youngest daughter. "She's a picky eater, so that's what I have to do." Both parents admitted they were getting a little worried for her as well.

I said, "Do you want two obese daughters? Because she is going to get there too." I looked at both parents to see if I had their attention. They looked uncomfortable. "Actually, it is the two of you that are responsible for Nicky's weight. She is only fourteen. She doesn't have any income to purchase the food that she eats. She relies solely on the decisions that you, her parents, make. Yes, she is responsible for how much she puts in her mouth, but she will eat what you provide." This stopped the blame game between them and pointed everyone in the same direction toward helping Nicky.

I made some suggestions for changes, such as having zero-calorie beverages and almond milk for Nicky (which she loved). I pointed out the savings from purchasing fewer unhealthy snacks and replacing them with healthier snacks, such as nuts and fruits. One less each of a bag of chips, a package of cookies, and container of fruit juice would save about $10 per shopping trip. The mother said she liked the idea of saving money. I pointed out that it can be more expensive to be overweight and unhealthy than to maintain a healthy weight. I was encouraged when the mother leaned back, patted her own stomach, and said, "You think I could get rid of this?"

The problem was not a Nicky problem, but a family problem. As we talked, I saw greater understanding on the parents' faces. I suggested that the parents have some joint sessions with Nicky and the psychiatrist. Toward the end of our discussion, I asked if she felt that I had given her some ideas and tools to help her lose weight and she said she did. Most importantly, her parents understood the need to change.

Parents need to consider their own shopping and eating habits for the sake of their children's health. When the child gains weight, the blame is sometimes placed on fast food restaurants, school lunches—and worse—the child. Even when the child attempts to do something about it, as in Nicky's case, their attempts will fail if they don't get the right kind of support from their parents. As these children grow into obese adults, the parents throw their hands up and say that they tried, or the child wouldn't listen. Yet, everything starts in the home.

Children who witness the resentment between their parents and blame themselves don't always know how to express their desperation and may express themselves in inappropriate ways or self-harm. Nicky's parents were very good at arguing and complaining about her eating too much, but they were never able to teach her what healthy foods to eat or proper serving sizes were. Why? Because they never knew what a serving was or how to count calories and they didn't understand much about shopping for healthy foods.

Become Actively Involved

I have seen and heard of parents who lash out at medical professionals when they are told their child is overweight or obese. Or they *fire* their child's pediatrician when the pediatrician tells them their child needs to lose weight. Another example is when an upset parent calls the school and yells at the teachers for sending home a BMI report indicating that their child is obese. These parents are angry at the physician or the school for being insensitive and embarrassing their child. Yet, it was the parents who set their child up for embarrassment in the first place. Such parents are modeling the victim mentality that we discussed in an earlier chapter.

Every child needs an adult to guide them. Everything that we, as parents, do or say, does not go unnoticed by our children. A good example of this comes from my friend's son, Jeramiah, who is ten years old. He told me a story about a recent health class at his school. The entire class had done so well on their tests that the new principal came by and praised them. She then gave them all rewards that were coupons for a small smoothie from a major fast food restaurant. Jeramiah was curious and looked online for the nutrition data. He found out that the smoothies had almost 300 calories and over 50 grams of sugar. He thought it was ironic that the authority figure was handing these out in the middle of a health class without a second thought. From the principal's point of view, giving coupons was a nice thing to do, and a lot cheaper than giving every student a bicycle. Yet, the best reward for these children was the knowledge of healthy eating.

The difference between Jeramiah and Nicky is that Jeramiah's parents are more knowledgeable about health and nutrition. The incident with the principal simply becomes a joke in Jeramiah's family. He can have a frank discussion at home and can hold his own at school without a need to call out the principal, who was well meaning, but not thinking things through. Jeramiah's parents also had no need to make an ugly phone call to the principal or shame her on social media. They had no desire to turn a sincere, but misplaced gesture into something dramatic. They were on solid ground. On the other hand, Nicky has no one to turn to because her parents are not as informed, or as involved as Jeramiah's parents. Nicky had no one to guide her. She was encouraged to eat poorly, because her parents failed to know what was right or wrong. When parents fail to be accountable for their actions, they blame others, like the school, the restaurant, or even their pediatrician, deflecting, misdirecting and modeling the wrong behavior for the child. We have to wonder how Nicky will handle life challenges, as an adult, compared to Jeramiah.

Home Is Where It All Begins

The warmth of the relationship among family members forms an inseparable bond. Parents' unconditional love for their children is the most powerful force necessary for children to develop a feeling of security and confidence. Within the family, the needs of different family members can create complex dynamics leading to struggles within the family. Sometimes, we forget that the people our children watch and copy the most are us. When we divert the blame to someone else, or blame the child for their actions, it causes a lot of confusion in their young, developing minds.

Parents are in the driver's seat for creating healthy eating habits and building their children's knowledge about food. They need to "drive the bus." It doesn't help if they drive off in the wrong direction and all end up in the wrong place. Parents need to take the time and commit to planning for meals and purchasing the right foods. Just like they need to find time to exercise and have fun as a family and create balance in their lives. Simply ask yourself: What can I do so that we, as a family don't become a burden to each other and so that we can have a happy life together? Your answer and your desire to be free from burden may be your motivation to lose weight, among the many other reasons that you have learned from reading this book.

15. Keeping It Off = Longevity

"If a person knows "what" happens, they have average ability;

If they know "how" it happens, they have superior ability;

If they know "why" it happens, they have exceptional ability."

Marilyn vos Savant

The quote above was by a writer and lecturer, someone knowledgeable about many subjects. She is also known for having the highest recorded IQ ever. Her quote is a great way to sum up the journey through this book. In the beginning, we learned about obesity and its effects. We learned about *what* happens to the body when it consumes too much food. When we become aware of how our environment influences us, we learn about *how* it happens. We also recognize *why* it is very important to develop a certain state of awareness to successfully manage our weight. Even with this knowledge, the journey can be challenging. If there is one thing that is more frustrating than the struggle to lose weight, it is the challenge of keeping it off.

When a person loses weight, metabolic and hormonal changes can counteract their efforts. The body fights against weight loss. Because of these changes and the physiological resetting of the body's energy thermostat, people who lose weight will have difficulty keeping the weight off.

Changes to our metabolism can be significant. For example, a person weighing 250 pounds loses 30 pounds, a little over 10% of their weight. Changes to their metabolism means they must either eat fewer calories a day than someone who had always been 220 pounds, or they need to exercise more to maintain this new weight. The basal metabolic rate (BMR) calculators online do not account for weight loss conditions, therefore anyone taking part in a weight-loss plan needs to be aware of this fact or else they will plateau or gain the weight back.

A good example of this was found in a scientific research study[1] performed on contestants of the famous TV show "The Biggest Loser." Of the 16 contestants, only one continued to lose weight after the show was done filming. All of the others had gained most, if not all of their weight back that they had lost during the show. Some gained more. Why, and how can this happen? These people had world-class coaches and nutritional guidance, yet still gained all their weight back. One reason why they gained it all back is because of metabolic changes in the body due to weight loss.

The metabolic rate of an obese person is normal for their weight prior to weight loss and decreases substantially as they lose weight. This process causes metabolic stress that can continue for years. Even more fascinating is that the metabolic rates never stabilize to the level of others who are at the same weight, but have not had substantial weight loss. The "Biggest Losers" were performing an uphill battle against their own biology. Because of this, some eventually had bariatric surgery or additional therapeutic methods of weight control.

A reality show setting, especially when teams are competing under intense public scrutiny, is very different from the home environment. After the 30 weeks of strenuous diet and exercise, each contestant must go home to their pre-show environment and families. It is speculation to wonder what challenges the contestants had faced prior to the show that they had to go back to once the show was over in addition to dealing with the inherent struggle because of the change in body weight.

In another study on weight-loss[2], researchers followed over 400 people for five years after their weight loss surgery. The weight loss in the beginning was significant with most of the participants losing up to 77% of their excess weight in the first year. Yet, during the next five years, they regained about half of their original weight[3]. One of the study physicians described weight-loss surgery as an attempt at "behavioral surgery" since people who did not change their behavior would regain their weight.

The idea of weight-loss surgery is to change the size and function of the gastrointestinal tract, yet *the true target is the brain*. The imposition of a physical restraint on the stomach, having surgery, is a way to allow people to retrain their minds, but an overwhelming majority of people fail to change their desires and behaviors for the long term. In each chapter of this book, we saw where some of the most difficult challenges are in our everyday lives. The next example is about Henry, who kept the weight off after surgery, but admitted that it wasn't as easy as he had thought.

Henry: Keeping It off after Surgery

The first time I met Henry, I would never have guessed that he had been morbidly obese until he told me about his gastric bypass surgery and how he had lost a lot of weight. During his time in the Air Force, he stayed fit because of his military routine and his environment. He gained all his weight after he retired; the dramatic change in his routine was a direct cause for his morbid obesity.

During our first meeting at a Mexican restaurant, I noticed how he was eating tortilla chips. He was breaking each chip into smaller pieces before scooping up the salsa. And I thought I was the only one that did that to regulate carbs. Henry later explained that he had to dramatically change the way he ate, because there was a time when he could have died if he didn't change his lifestyle.

A few years after he retired, he had gained a tremendous amount of weight. He was 5 feet 9 inches tall and weighed about 285 pounds with a BMI of 42.1 and had type 2 diabetes. He attributed it to losing the structure and active lifestyle required in the military. When he maxed out on oral diabetic medications his endocrinologist put him on an insulin pump. Even then, his diabetes was difficult to control, and he was going through a vial of insulin every few days.

His mother was also diabetic. One day, when she was in her garden, she stuck her foot on a thorn from her rose bush and it quickly became infected. The wound would not heal, and her foot had to be amputated. Even after this the infection continued, and her surgeons had to amputate her leg just below the knee. Modern medicine could not save his mother's leg.

This was Henry's wake-up call. He decided it was time for a change. At a weight-loss support meeting, he saw the drastic before and after pictures of people who had undergone weight loss surgery and heard their stories. After he went through the necessary tests that included a psychiatric evaluation, he had a successful gastric bypass surgery. The early results were dramatic. He dropped approximately 10 pounds even while he was still in the hospital and another 10-15 pounds within the week after his discharge. He was still diabetic, but his insulin requirement was now minimal.

"Those early days were hard," he said. "Every time I wanted to overeat, I would get clogged up in my head. I had to change my mind to recognize that I was not going to starve to death." He had to train himself to stop eating. He had to make the right choices and never overeat.

He continued to describe his thoughts on how he overcame food addiction. "I had to learn how to chew. I would watch my wife, my family, and my friends. They chew only a few times and swallow their food. For me, it takes a little longer because I chew a lot. I feel that when I do it, I get the food to a consistency that's easier for my body to digest. I also get to taste the food a little longer." This comment reminded me about the method of mindful eating discussed earlier. He shared a story about going to the mall with his wife shortly after the surgery. They went to a fast food restaurant and ordered small milk shakes. "I had barely sipped a quarter of the shake when I started feeling nauseous. That's when I knew that my body was processing food in an entirely different way than before."

We talked about the folds of skin and fat that accompany the weight loss. He admitted that the folds did appear, but it didn't bother him too much. "I used to lift up my arms and the skin would hang down," he said. "But now, I can lift my arms and there is no loose skin. I'm older. I'm happily married. That's more important than tight skin." He explained how the skin shrank over several years and did conform to his body shape.

Henry walked regularly for exercise and played softball with friends, but he didn't belong to a gym. During the summer, he is more active and drops another 10 pounds. His surgery was 12 years ago, and today he weighs around 180 pounds with a BMI of 26.6 and still diabetic. Although he no longer uses insulin, he takes a newer medicine that comes as a weekly injection. Some days his blood glucose is around 101, which is as close to a non-diabetic person's fasting glucose level as it can be.

I asked him what advice he would give to people who wanted to keep the weight off. He was kind enough to share some insights:

| Food is always there for you, but it can also hurt you. It's about changing your mind set, the way you deal with food. |
| When I go out, I tell the waiter to give me just half a portion. If they can't, I always ask for a box and take half of my food home. |
| He drinks alcohol, but less than what he used to. One glass of wine or beer will give him a good buzz. If he orders a beer, he makes it lasts for at least a half-hour. |
| Don't worry about the loose skin folds or how your body looks. Worry about losing weight. |

Is Henry just lucky, or is he an anomaly, like that one person out of all the contestants in the reality show? I don't think so, because of what I know about Henry and his environment. He and his wife, Jenny, agree on most things, including food. Also, there is not one spouse getting upset with the other about who is losing weight faster than the other. Jenny takes care of herself, watches what she eats, and maintains a healthy BMI. Not only do their zones of influences overlap—they are complementary. Henry seems to have achieved the happiness, freedom, and peace of mind that we discussed at the beginning of the book.

Weight Loss Surgery: Not an Instant Solution

We live in a society where we want convenience, an instant solution, and one that lasts. While it is evident that the surgery can indeed deliver, most people cannot change the environment they live in. As I described throughout the book, how we interact with our environment affects our ability to lose weight. The same challenge remains after the initial weight loss because although you have changed, your surroundings have not.

People who choose weight-loss surgery must have a thorough psychiatric evaluation before the procedure. They are instructed to adopt healthy eating habits before and after the surgery. I believe that long-term success like Henry's could be enjoyed by more people regardless of whether they lose weight with diet, medications, or surgery, if they bear in mind that they must have a plan to deal with their environment, as well as their family relationships.

Food is integral to our survival, but also helps us nurture, celebrate, grieve, retreat, overcome, and emerge. Weight management and certain metabolic diseases are areas where man-made drugs and surgery cannot always overcome the human will and emotion. Therefore, a long-term weight management strategy cannot simply be about food, but must consider our very nature and humanity.

Sometimes, this means dealing with the fact that not everyone has the same priorities or expectations as you have. This includes close family members who love you and long-time friends but have no interest in adopting a healthy lifestyle. It can be a challenge to live with them, but being aware of when your boundaries are being breached will let you manage such situations with confidence.

Weight Loss Is a Marathon, Not a Sprint

Even under the best of circumstances, life is not easy, and with our increased life expectancy, we can expect it to be a long journey. Overweight and obesity usually start on a clean slate, that is, we are of normal weight before becoming overweight and obese. Before the weight begins to add up, we have an inherent potential for a long and healthy life. Regardless of our weight, our chances of getting different illnesses increase with time and age, merely from being on this earth. But when we become overweight or obese, it creates an additional risk on top of what we would naturally experience. Not one of us set out on our life journey with the goal of turning our bodies into bags of medicine from having to treat chronic diseases caused by our weight.

Here is a story from the Buddha's life that is a good example of what I'm trying to say. During Buddha's travels, he encountered a woman crying and grieving over the recent death of her son. He had died of a snake bite and Buddha said to the woman, "I will grant you one wish. I will give you either a pot of gold or your son's life back." The woman quickly responded, "I would like to have my son bring me a pot of gold." This is the Burmese version of "Have your cake and eat it too." Life is a one-way street and we are all on this journey together. Why settle for anything less than all that life has to offer? In the preceding chapters, we discussed the different things that can distract us and make us forget that we are on a journey. Although it is important to know what caused us to gain weight, it is even more important to decide how we will manage our weight loss in the long run.

Here is some advice from Tony Robbins, the well-known life coach and entrepreneur: "Want to learn to eat a lot? Eat a little. That way, you will be around long enough to eat a lot." In the race for longevity, the last person to cross the finish line gets to eat the most. In this particular journey, the ones in the slow lane are the winners. They take it all.

Design a Routine that Works for You.

The martial arts legend, Bruce Lee, described his philosophy of doing more with less:

When we allow ourselves to be distracted by the latest fad diets and supplements, follow quick-fix diet experts, we allow ourselves to be distracted from what is important. One way to avoid distractions is through planning and routines. Having a routine seems boring, but it gives you control through discipline, consistency, and simplicity.

There are tech moguls who wear black turtle neck sweaters or grey t-shirts every day. Perhaps it is a signature style for them, or perhaps it is because they would rather focus on more important things. I like that we wear dark blue or grey scrubs at work, which takes the guesswork out of deciding my outfit each morning. When there is even one less "mundane" thing to worry about, it frees up your mind for other things because you have just brought simplicity to an element of your life.

Do you remember that I wrote about how we get stuck in certain routines that were convenient, and made us comfortable, but were not necessarily good for our waistlines? Well, we can turn the same principle around and apply it to managing our weight. A strategy that I have seen that works well is when people bring pre-measured portions of low-carb food for breakfast, lunch and snacks to work. Some make several portions of proteins and vegetables over the weekend and measure the portions into containers so that during the week, they can simply "grab and go." Another woman was very successful in keeping the weight off. When I asked her how she did it, she gave me a one-word answer, "Salad!" Each time she started gaining a few pounds, she started eating portion-controlled salads until she went back to her baseline. And by salad, she wasn't talking about pasta, potato, macaroni, or bean salads.

Several people I know stay on proteins and green vegetables during the week and ease their restrictions on the weekend. Others eat no, or low carbs for breakfast and dinner, opting to have their carbs for lunch. Let's face it, carbs are delicious and comforting, and with careful planning and choosing whole grain options, we can still enjoy moderate amounts of carbs as long as we plan for it.

Some people use a method along these lines to get ahead financially. They take advantage of automated deductions from their paychecks to contribute to their 401ks to bring discipline to investing. Warren Buffet, the renowned investor, has a simple way of starting out his day. Before driving to work each morning, he sets the budget for his McDonald's breakfast based on how the financial markets performed the previous day. If the market did well, he spends $3.17, if it didn't he spends $2.61 on set items, eliminating the need for guessing how much to spend, leaving his mind and day free to focus on other things that matter. Since he likes McDonald's the need to think about where to get breakfast becomes a non-issue. I'm not implying that Mr. Buffet couldn't afford more or became rich by saving on breakfast, but to make a point that establishing routines brings benefits to your life such as managing your weight and even beyond that. You may not become as wealthy, but with some planning and automation, you could trim your waistline while saving some money. This example shows that discipline can become effortless through forming habits.

Small Corrections Are Easier Than Major Ones

There are lessons we can learn from traveling to other countries that can apply to our journey through weight loss and maintenance. I read an article written by a woman who traveled to Asia on her own[4]. While she traveled to Hong Kong, a friend suggested an excursion to Japan. But once they got to Kyoto, she found herself alone after they had a disagreement and parted ways. She discovered the helpfulness of strangers who came to her assistance when she couldn't read the train schedules, find the tourist attractions, and didn't know the correct change for fares. After this, she encountered the furious pace of Tokyo, and could not find her way out of the gigantic Ikebukero train station for an hour. Once she got to her hotel, she decided that she would not put herself in a similar situation again and decided to *"Stay close and get lost small."*

As mentioned earlier, we see some people lose a lot of weight, only to regain it. It's important to know that in the medical management of obesity it's expected and accepted that people may regain some of their initial weight. As long as people don't exceed their original weight, it's not considered a failure. Sir Winston Churchill said it best when he said, "Success is not final, and failure is not fatal."

But when people regain large amounts of weight, it's possible that they had lost their "bearings." Small and prompt corrections are necessary when you are trying to maintain your new weight. Losing the few pounds of weight as soon as they are gained, will always be easier than waiting until you have gained twenty or thirty pounds, like the expression by the traveler in the example.

Just as landmarks and signs are useful in traveling around a city, our landmarks for maintaining weight loss are tools such as our scales, BMI and BMR. Small corrections to your habits and lifestyle are much easier than major ones.

Last Thoughts

So how much should we give credit to food when it comes to dieting? Let's review. In the earlier chapters, I discussed people's frustration with dieting and failing. We talked about creating a mindset for success, drawing on our past and orienting our minds to set the stage for the future. Chapter 4 described emotional eating and how we turn to food for comfort, then discussed how environmental factors affect food consumption. Then, we talked about setting boundaries and protecting our territories, as strategies for success. We examined how we calculate and manipulate things in our environment as a matter of daily survival tactics, and how we can apply this to calorie counting, therefore creating better boundaries.

I described in the Medications chapter and Weight chapter how our will power can sometimes be stronger than drugs and medicine. Our mindsets determine whether we use appetite suppressants successfully, and weight loss surgery had less to do with the stomach, but everything to do with the mind. We also discussed how we can keep our guard up against the way alcohol influences us, making us smarter consumers. Chapter 10 described how our perceptions are being guided by advertisements and the food industry, how they can manipulate our self-image, as well as our perception of others. The next chapter was about how we can get caught between the needs of loved ones, and how we sometimes unintentionally hurt the people we love. The final chapter has some suggestions about planning to keep the weight off, and how consciously structuring our life can give you freedom and power.

In reality, food has less to do with how we become overweight or obese, and more to do with our minds and how we manage ourselves around food and other influences. The same is true of keeping the weight off. Charles Darwin said, "It is not the strongest of the species that survives, nor the most intelligent one. It is the one that is most adaptable to change." Being adaptable, and understanding why things are the way they are, lets us enjoy the best that life has to offer.

Resources

Introduction

Why I wrote this book

1. https://en.wikipedia.org/wiki/The_Matrix

The Named Diets

1. http://www.consultant360.com/articles/todays-diets-do-they-work-fact-versus-fiction
2. https://en.wikipedia.org/wiki/Atkins_diet
3. http://jamanetwork.com/journals/jama/fullarticle/1900510
4. http://www.tandfonline.com/doi/full/10.1080/07315724.2017.1302367
5. https://en.wikipedia.org/wiki/Gluten-free_diet
6. http://www.aafp.org/afp/2014/0115/p82.html#afp20140115p82-b7
7. https://en.wikipedia.org/wiki/Non-celiac_gluten_sensitivity
8. http://journals.plos.org/plosone/article?id=10.1371/journal.pone.0175149
9. https://www.nhlbi.nih.gov/news/press-releases/2009/heart-healthy-reduced-calorie-diets-promote-long-term-weight-loss

Chapter 1

1. https://www.unce.unr.edu/publications/files/hn/2010/fs1011.pdf
2. http://jamanetwork.com/journals/jama/article-abstract/2553448
3. https://www.nhlbi.nih.gov/health/resources/heart/cholesterol-tlc

Chapter 2

1. http://www.medscape.com/viewarticle/806566.
2. Practice Guidelines: ADA Updated Standards of Medical Care for Patients with Diabetes Mellitus; American Family Physician, Volume 95, Number 1 January 1, 2017.

3. Published source: Diabetes Care, January 2016;39 (suppl): S1-S112.
4. http://www.webmd.com/heart/metabolic-syndrome/metabolic-syndrome-what-is-it#1
5. http://www.arthritis.org/living-with-arthritis/comorbidities/obesity-arthritis/fat-and-arthritis.php,
6. https://academic.oup.com/jnci/article/105/24/1907/2517573/Human-Gut-Microbiome-and-Risk-for-Colorectal

Chapter 3

1. https://www.linkedin.com/learning/powerless-to-powerful-taking-control/welcome
2. https://www.psychologytoday.com/blog/thriving101/201506/weight-loss-motivation-secrets-staying-track-part-1
3. http://changingminds.org/explanations/motivation/four_motivations.htm
4. http://www.stephencovey.com/blog/?tag=albert-e-n-gray

Chapter 4

1. https://www.ncbi.nlm.nih.gov/pmc/articles/PMC3486959/
2. http://www.nctsn.org/sites/default/files/assets/pdfs/SAToolkit_1.pdf
3. https://allpsych.com/journal/phobias/
4. https://www.ncbi.nlm.nih.gov/pmc/articles/PMC3124340/

Chapter 5

1. https://www.cdc.gov/bam/teachers/documents/epi_1_triangle.pdf
2. http://newsroom.heart.org/news/eating-in-social-settings-may-be-greatest-temptation-for-dieters

Chapter 6

1. https://www.justjohncrowley.com/how-i-quit-drinking-and-blew-up-my-sales-career/

Chapter 7

1. https://www.nhlbi.nih.gov/health/educational/lose_wt/eat/fd_exch.htm
2. https://www.nhlbi.nih.gov/health/educational/wecan/downloads/servingcard7.pdf
3. https://en.wikipedia.org/wiki/Sugar_alcohol

Chapter 8

1. http://www.webmd.com/diet/features/is-it-better-to-be-a-vegetarian

Chapter 9

1. https://www.nhlbi.nih.gov/health/educational/lose_wt/BMI/bmi-m.htm
2. https://www.acefitness.org/acefit/healthy-living-article/60/112/what-are-the-guidelines-for-percentage-of-body-fat
3. http://ajcn.nutrition.org/content/87/5/1212.full
4. https://www.nhlbi.nih.gov/health/educational/lose_wt/risk.htm
5. http://www.fao.org/docrep/007/y5686e/y5686e09.htm
6. http://www.active.com/fitness/calculators/calories

Chapter 10

1. https://www.cdc.gov/physicalactivity/basics/adults/index.htm
2. https://www.livescience.com/32475-why-do-we-shiver-when-cold.htmlhen
3. https://www.medpagetoday.com/Endocrinology/Obesity/66272?xid=nl_mpt_DHE_2017-06-27&eun=g653965d0r&pos=2
4. http://newsnetwork.mayoclinic.org/discussion/mayo-clinic-discovers-high-intensity-aerobic-training-can-reverse-aging-processes-in-adults/
5. http://www.cnn.com/2017/03/06/health/cardio-lifting-weight-loss-partner/

Chapter 11

1. http://science.sciencemag.org/content/306/5695/457
2. https://www.sciencedaily.com/releases/2014/08/140825185319.htm
3. http://www.consultant360.com/articles/initiating-injectable-treatment-type-2-diabetes-focus-glucagon-peptide-1-receptor-agonists
4. https://www.niaaa.nih.gov/alcohol-health/overview-alcohol-consumption/moderate-binge-drinking

Chapter 12

1. https://www.livestrong.com/article/294819-how-many-calories-does-one-gram-of-alcohol-equal/
2. https://answers.webmd.com/answers/1166926/how-is-alcohol-metabolized
3. http://www.usatoday.com/story/news/health/2013/10/29/alcohol-no-nutrition-labels/3305395/
4. http://www.culinarylore.com/drinks:meaning-of-proof-and-measuring-alcohol-amount
5. https://medlineplus.gov/ency/patientinstructions/000886.htm
6. https://www.rethinkingdrinking.niaaa.nih.gov/Tools/Calculators/calorie-calculator.aspx

Chapter 13

1. https://www.ncbi.nlm.nih.gov/pmc/articles/PMC3234679/
2. http://www.nhs.uk/news/2015/07July/Pages/are-overweight-teens-unaware-of-their-size.aspx
3. http://www.ajpmonline.org/article/S0749-3797(15)00146-4/fulltext
4. http://jamanetwork.com/journals/jama/article-abstract/2643761
5. https://www.cancer.org/cancer/cancer-causes/diet-physical-activity/body-weight-and-cancer-risk/effects.html
6. http://www.medscape.com/viewarticle/874311
7. https://www.britannica.com/science/somatotype

Chapter 14

1. http://www.medscape.com/viewarticle/710209_2
2. http://jamanetwork.com/journals/jamapediatrics/fullarticle/485676
3. https://www.cdc.gov/nchs/ppt/nchs2012/ss-32_claassen.pdf

Chapter 15

1. http://onlinelibrary.wiley.com/doi/10.1002/oby.21538/full
2. http://jamanetwork.com/journals/jamasurgery/fullarticle/2422341
3. https://consumer.healthday.com/vitamins-and-nutrition-information-27/dieting-to-lose-weight-health-news-195/weight-loss-surgery-s-benefits-may-fade-with-time-study-suggests-702043.html
4. http://www.oprah.com/world/traveling-to-japan-alone-overcoming-shyness

Tips for Shopping

1. http://www.mass.gov/eohhs/gov/departments/dph/programs/community-health/mass-in-motion/kids-health/eat-better/grocery-shopping.html
2. https://www.choosemyplate.gov/

Many supermarkets arrange their aisles in a fairly consistent way[1]. Produce, meat, seafood, poultry, the deli, bakery, dairy products and eggs, frozen foods, are arranged around the perimeter. Canned goods, starches, soda, snacks and other items are found in the center. The easiest way to shop for healthy foods is to shop around the perimeter of the supermarket.

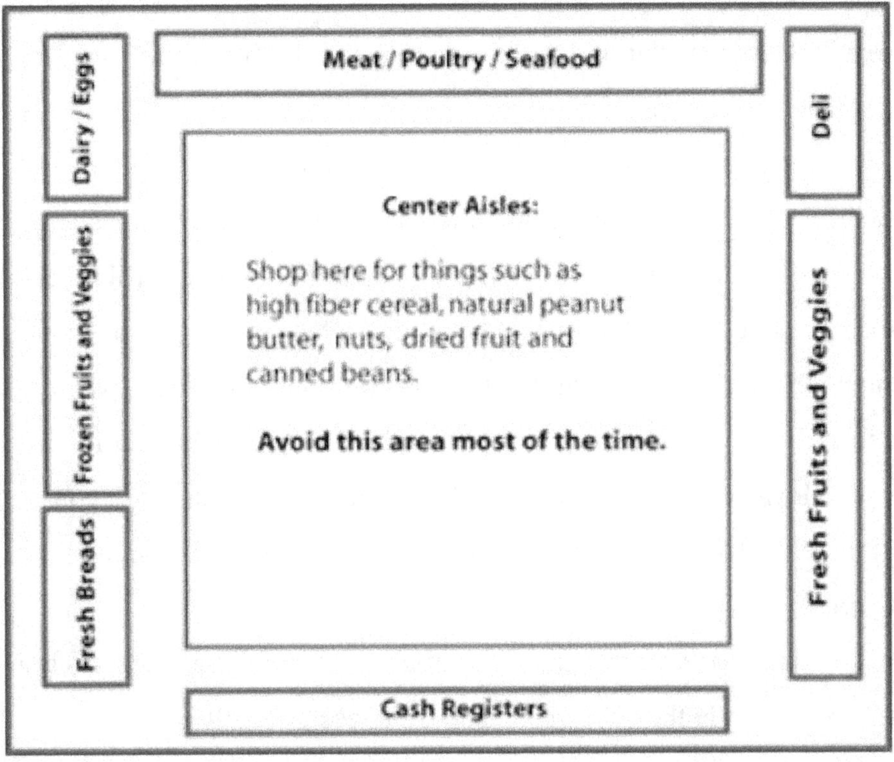

The produce section will have a variety of vegetables and fruits. Produce has the fewest number of calories and include: leafy greens, such as spinach, lettuce, and herbs, and other vegetables such as onions, peppers, broccoli, Brussel sprouts, cabbage and green beans. Not all greens are created equal. Green peas and lima beans[2] are considered starchy vegetables and are in the same food group as corn, potatoes, sweet potatoes, yams. Fruits become sweeter and their glycemic index increases as they ripen. Among fruits, avocados provide a good source of healthy fats.

The meat and seafood section offer high quality proteins. They have no carbs and the number of calories depends on the type of meat. Some have a higher in fat than others, and too much saturated fat, such as the fat found in red meat, can be bad for your heart health. Remember to take a look at the nutrition label to see how the servings are divided, types of fat, and cholesterol.

In the dairy section, eggs are the cheapest, complete source of protein. At one time, it was thought to cause high levels of the bad cholesterol, LDL, but new research shows that LDL cholesterol levels have more to do with how our bodies process fats and not so much the fat content of foods. Greek yogurt has a higher amount of protein when compared to regular or low-fat yogurt and will suppress hunger much longer. However, when granola is added, both calories and carb content will increase. Cheese, including cottage cheese, is a good source of protein.

Some frozen foods are great time savers. Frozen vegetables are flash frozen while they are fresh. The packages typically have just one ingredient listed. Frozen meals, while they are a quick solution to our busy schedules, can be high in sodium and preservatives. On the other hand, these are useful as a guide to see what one meal portion should look like, along with the corresponding caloric count. As you can see, if you were to put the frozen meal on a plate, it is much smaller than a restaurant entrée, or what many people typically think of as a portion. But, they are still filling, and will hold us till the next meal. Take a trip down this aisle to read the nutrition labels on the various frozen meals and you will see the ingredients in the low carb meals. They are mostly meat and vegetables. Sometimes, the meals with pasta will contain soy protein that is a complete protein. For those who are not inclined to weigh and measure ingredients, frozen meals are a quick way to learn about portion sizes and calories in a portion of a cooked meal, and this knowledge can be applied when cooking at home and when eating at restaurants.

When shopping in the center of the store, one of the smartest things you can do is to read the nutrition labels as described in the chapter on calorie counting. Center aisles do offer some healthy items such as nuts, peanut butter, and whole grains. If you read the nutrition labels on some of the whole grain breads, there are still a fair amount of net carbs after the fiber is subtracted. However, even small amounts of fiber can help you feel full longer.

Here are some other things to consider, especially when there is a need to keep items in stock. Canned vegetables contain few ingredients other than the vegetables themselves and water. They also vary in their carbohydrate content and most canned soups contain two servings.

The aisle with the baking ingredients may seem scary, but there are several types of artificial sweeteners to eliminate the need for calories from sugar. There has been controversy around the effect of these sweeteners on weight, but just like many studies, there are other factors that may affect the study itself. Moderation is key.

Whole grains and lentils provide a good source of fiber. Lentils provide some protein, but both have somewhat higher levels of carbs than animal proteins or soy.

Try to keep visits to the bakery as infrequent as possible and save them for special occasions. What about the cake on the cover? I ate it—

over a period of a month—in small pieces, and it was very good. And you can do the same. Most bakery items store well in the freezer, so there is no reason to eat it all in one setting.

The recipes in the next section are low in carbohydrates, starting with a very simple recipe as an example to show one serving with very few ingredients.

Breakfast Recipes

Classic Bacon and Eggs

Ingredients:

2 large eggs

3 slices Bacon

Salt

Pepper

Directions:

1. In a medium sized pan, heat bacon to desired crispness on medium-high heat. Flip when necessary.
2. Remove bacon from pan when it is finished and set on paper towel lined plate.
3. Pour out majority of bacon grease leaving a little bit in the pan (about ½ a tbsp.) Enough to cover the bottom.
4. Crack eggs into pan and fry in the bacon grease until cooked to desired doneness.
5. Season with salt and pepper.

Nutrition Facts	
Servings 1.0	
Amount Per Serving	
Calories 263	
	% Daily Value*
Total Fat 19g	28%
Saturated Fat 7g	34%
Monounsaturated Fat 4g	
Polyunsaturated Fat 2g	
Trans Fat 0 g	
Cholesterol 402 mg	134%
Sodium 667 mg	28%
Potassium 138 mg	4%
Total Carbohydrate 1g	0%
Fiber 0 g	0%
Sugars 0 g	
Protein 22 g	43%
Vitamin A	11%
Vitamin C	0%
Calcium	6%
Iron	13%

*Based on a 2,000 calorie diet, your values may be different. Values may not be 100% accurate, and have not been evaluated professionally or by the US FDA.

Vegetable Breakfast Skillet

Ingredients:

1 Green Bell Pepper

1 Red Bell Pepper

2 cups Mushrooms

1 dash Salt

1 dash black pepper

1 cup shredded, Cheese, cheddar

8 large eggs

1/3 cup Onion

Cooking Spray

Directions:

1. In a large bowl beat eggs until well blended.
2. Slice peppers, mushrooms, and onion into thin strips.
3. In a large pan on medium-high heat, spray with cooking spray and sauté vegetables until tender. Remove and set aside.
4. Turn the pan down to low and spray with cooking spray again.
5. Pour eggs into pan and continuously stir until it begins to clump up.
6. Once the eggs are almost cooked, add the vegetables back into the pan and fold into the eggs.
7. Add the cheese and stir it into the eggs until melted and incorporated.
8. Add salt and pepper to taste.

Nutrition Facts	
Servings 4.0	
Amount Per Serving	
Calories 302	
	% Daily Value*
Total Fat 21 g	32%
Saturated Fat 10 g	48%
Monounsaturated Fat 6 g	
Polyunsaturated Fat 2 g	
Trans Fat 0 g	
Cholesterol 406 mg	135%
Sodium 430 mg	18%
Potassium 244 mg	7%
Total Carbohydrate 6 g	2%
Fiber 2 g	9%
Sugars 3 g	
Protein 22 g	44%
Vitamin A	36%
Vitamin C	65%
Calcium	29%
Iron	12%

*Based on a 2,000 calorie diet, your values may be different. Values may not be 100% accurate, and have not been evaluated professionally or by the US FDA.

Southern Style Drop Biscuits and Sausage Gravy

Ingredients:

1/2 tsp. Baking Soda (leavening agent)
1/4 tsp. Sea Salt, salt, pepper
1/4 cup Stevia in the Raw
2 tbsp. Unsweetened Almond Milk
6 tbsp. Egg, whites only
1/4 tsp. Apple Cider Vinegar
2 cups Unsweetened Almond Milk
½ tbsp. Xanthan Gum
3 tbsp. coconut oil (melted, can sub for butter)
2 cups Blanched Almond Flour
8 oz. Jimmy Dean - Country Mild Sausage, cooked

Directions:

1. Preheat oven to 350 degrees.
2. In a large bowl, combine almond flour, baking soda, salt, and stevia and mix well.
3. In another bowl, combine 2 tbsp. almond milk, egg whites, and apple cider vinegar.
4. Combine the liquid and dry ingredients together and mix well.
5. On a parchment or silicone lined baking pan, drop six evenly sized dollops onto the pan about two inches apart.
6. Bake the biscuits for about 15 minutes or until golden brown.
7. While the biscuits are baking, brown sausage in a medium-sized pan on medium-high heat.
8. Remove sausage and set aside leaving the drippings in the pan.
9. Add almond milk to the pan and begin stirring with a whisk.
10. Slowly incorporate xanthan gum, sprinkling it in while stirring until a thicker consistency is achieved. The entire ½ tablespoon may not be needed.
11. Add salt and pepper to taste and stir in the cooked sausage.
12. Serve warm biscuits with gravy.

Nutrition Facts	
Servings 8.0	
Amount Per Serving	
Calories 299	
% Daily Value*	
Total Fat 28 g	44%
Saturated Fat 9 g	
Monounsaturated Fat 1 g	
Polyunsaturated Fat 0 g	
Trans Fat 0 g	
Cholesterol 18 mg	6%
Sodium 454 mg	19%
Potassium 9 mg	0%
Total Carbohydrate 8 g	3%
Fiber 4 g	15%
Sugars 2 g	
Protein 13 g	26%
Vitamin A	4%
Vitamin C	0%
Calcium	19%
Iron	7%

*Based on a 2,000 calorie diet, your values may be different. Values may not be 100% accurate, and have not been evaluated professionally or by the US FDA.

Hot Sausage and Cheese Omelet

Ingredients:

3 tbsp. egg, white only

1 oz. Hot Breakfast Sausage

2 tbsp. shredded Cheese, cheddar

1 large egg

Salt and Pepper

Directions:

1. Beat egg and egg white together in a bowl.
2. In a small pan, brown and break sausage into crumbles over medium heat.
3. Pour eggs over browned sausage.
4. Once egg is starting to firm, carefully flip over.
5. Sprinkle shredded cheese over the egg and fold over on itself.

Nutrition Facts	
Servings 1.0	
Amount Per Serving	
Calories 309	
% Daily Value*	
Total Fat 23 g	35%
Saturated Fat 10 g	50%
Monounsaturated Fat 4 g	
Polyunsaturated Fat 1 g	
Trans Fat 0 g	
Cholesterol 237 mg	79%
Sodium 522 mg	22%
Potassium 165 mg	5%
Total Carbohydrate 2 g	
Fiber 0 g	0%
Sugars 1 g	
Protein 22 g	45%
Vitamin A	12%
Vitamin C	0%
Calcium	23%
Iron	6%

*Based on a 2,000 calorie diet, your values may be different. Values may not be 100% accurate, and have not been evaluated professionally or by the US FDA.

Crustless Spinach and Mushroom Quiche

Ingredients:

2 tbsp. Butter

1 tsp. Olive Oil

10 oz. Raw Spinach

8 oz. Mushroom

10 oz. Swiss Cheese, shredded

6 large eggs

1/2 cup Heavy Whipping Cream

1 dash Salt

½ tsp. Pepper

2/3 cup Onion, chopped

Directions:

1. Preheat oven to 400F.
2. In a large pan heat up olive oil and butter on medium heat and cook onions until translucent.
3. Add spinach (if fresh), mushrooms, and olives, and cook until the spinach is wilted.
4. Remove pan from heat and let cool while preparing the eggs.
5. In a large bowl, mix together eggs, heavy cream, salt, and pepper.
6. Gently add in the lukewarm vegetables to the bowl and stir in half the cheese.
7. Get a 9-inch pie or quiche pan and spray the inside with cooking spray.
8. Gently pour the mixture into the pan and spread evenly.
9. Sprinkle the remaining cheese on top of the quiche and place it in the oven.
10. Bake until puffed and golden brown, about 30 to 45 minutes, or until a toothpick stuck in the center comes out clean.
11. Let cool for 20 to 30 minutes before serving.

Nutrition Facts	
Servings 8.0	
Amount Per Serving	
Calories 278	
% Daily Value*	
Total Fat 22 g	34%
Saturated Fat 13 g	64%
Monounsaturated Fat 6 g	
Polyunsaturated Fat 1 g	
Trans Fat 0 g	
Cholesterol 200 mg	67%
Sodium 148 mg	6%
Potassium 135 mg	4%
Total Carbohydrate 4 g	1%
Fiber 1 g	2%
Sugars 2 g	
Protein 15 g	30%
Vitamin A	25%
Vitamin C	4%
Calcium	32%
Iron	5%

*Based on a 2,000 calorie diet, your values may be different. Values may not be 100% accurate, and have not been evaluated professionally or by the US FDA.

Scrambled Eggs and Smoked Salmon

Ingredients:

8 large eggs

1/4 lb. Fish, salmon, chinook, smoked and chopped into small sized pieces

1/4 cup Heavy Cream

2 tbsp. Butter

Salt

Pepper

1 tbsp. Raw Chives, chopped

Directions:

1. In a large bowl, beat together eggs and heavy cream until starting to foam.
2. In a large non-stick pan, melt butter over medium-low heat.
3. Add eggs and stir continuously with a rubber spatula until just beginning to firm up. They should still be semi-wet.
4. Add chopped salmon and gently fold into the eggs.
5. Sprinkle chives over the entire pan and season to taste with salt and pepper.

Nutrition Facts	
Servings 4.0	
Amount Per Serving	
Calories 277	
	% Daily Value*
Total Fat 20 g	30%
Saturated Fat 10 g	52%
Monounsaturated Fat 6 g	
Polyunsaturated Fat 2 g	
Trans Fat 0 g	
Cholesterol 414 mg	138%
Sodium 455 mg	19%
Potassium 205 mg	6%
Total Carbohydrate 1 g	0%
Fiber 0 g	0%
Sugars 0 g	
Protein 18 g	36%
Vitamin A	20%
Vitamin C	1%
Calcium	6%
Iron	12%

*Based on a 2,000 calorie diet, your values may be different. Values may not be 100% accurate, and have not been evaluated professionally or by the US FDA.

Quick Microwave Cinnamon Porridge

Ingredients:

2 tbsp. Raw Hemps Seeds, shelled

2 tbsp. Unsweetened Shredded Coconut

2 tbsp. Flaxseed Meal

1 tsp. Stevia in the Raw

Pinch of Salt

1 tsp. Cinnamon

1/2 tsp. Pure Vanilla Extract

1/2 cup Unsweetened Almond Milk

Directions:

1. Put all ingredients in a microwave safe bowl that is tall enough for a 2-inch gap between the mixture and the top of the bowl.
2. Microwave for 2 minutes stirring everything 30 seconds, or until thickened.

Nutrition Facts	
Servings 1.0	
Amount Per Serving	
Calories 299	
% Daily Value*	
Total Fat 26 g	40%
Saturated Fat 10 g	48%
Monounsaturated Fat 3g	
Polyunsaturated Fat 11 g	
Trans Fat 0 g	
Cholesterol 0 mg	0%
Sodium 199 mg	8%
Potassium 335 mg	10%
Total Carbohydrate 11 g	4%
Fiber 10 g	41%
Sugars 2 g	
Protein 11 g	22%
Vitamin A	5%
Vitamin C	0%
Calcium	26%
Iron	20%

*Based on a 2,000 calorie diet, your values may be different. Values may not be 100% accurate, and have not been evaluated professionally or by the US FDA.

Egg Muffin Frittatas

Ingredients:

6 large eggs

1/2 cup Milk

1/4 tsp. Salt

1/4 tsp. Pepper

1 cup Cheddar Cheese, shredded

1/4 cup Red Bell Pepper

1/4 cup Green Bell Pepper

1/3 cup Onion

1/2 lb. Cooked Breakfast Sausage (browned into crumbles)

Directions:

1. Preheat oven to 350F.
2. Chop bell peppers and onion into small pieces.
3. Beat together eggs, milk, salt, and pepper.
4. Mix together vegetables, cooked breakfast sausage, eggs, and half of the cheddar cheese.
5. Spray cooking spray over a 12-muffin cup baking pan.
6. Spoon mixture evenly into each of the tins.
7. Sprinkle the remaining cheese over each egg muffin.
8. Bake for about 20 minutes, or until set and the cheese has lightly browned.
9. Use the broiler for a few minutes to crisp the cheese if desired.

Nutrition Facts	
Servings 6.0	
Amount Per Serving	
Calories 283	
	% Daily Value*
Total Fat 21 g	33%
Saturated Fat 9 g	43%
Monounsaturated Fat 3 g	
Polyunsaturated Fat 1 g	
Trans Fat 0 g	
Cholesterol 235 mg	78%
Sodium 569 mg	24%
Potassium 159 mg	5%
Total Carbohydrate 4 g	1%
Fiber 1 g	3%
Sugars 2 g	
Protein 18 g	36%
Vitamin A	26%
Vitamin C	62%
Calcium	17%
Iron	7%

*Based on a 2,000 calorie diet, your values may be different. Values may not be 100% accurate, and have not been evaluated professionally or by the US FDA.

Apple Cinnamon Muffins

Ingredients:

1 tbsp. Ground Cinnamon

1 Medium Apple, cored and chopped into small pieces

1/2 tsp. baking soda (leavening agent)

1/4 tsp. Salt

1 tsp. Vanilla Extract

1 cup Coconut Flour

1/2 cup Unsalted Butter, melted

1 1/4 cup eggs, white only

3/4 cup Stevia in the Raw

Directions:

1. Preheat oven to 350 degrees F.
2. In a large bowl, mix together all dry ingredients thoroughly. (Leave out apples).
3. Add eggs into the mixture and fold in until fully incorporated.
4. Fold in apple pieces.
5. Spray a 12-cup muffin tin with cooking spray or grease with butter.
6. Spoon batter equally into each muffin cup.
7. Bake for 25 to 30 minutes, or until a toothpick inserted comes out clean.

NOTE: Serving size is 2 muffins.

Nutrition Facts	
Servings 6.0	
Amount Per Serving	
Calories 260	
	% Daily Value*
Total Fat 18 g	28%
Saturated Fat 12 g	62%
Monounsaturated Fat 4 g	
Polyunsaturated Fat 1 g	
Trans Fat 0 g	
Cholesterol 41 mg	14%
Sodium 305 mg	13%
Potassium 121 mg	3%
Total Carbohydrate 17 g	6%
Fiber 8 g	32%
Sugars 6 g	
Protein 8 g	17%
Vitamin A	10%
Vitamin C	1%
Calcium	3%
Iron	14%

*Based on a 2,000 calorie diet, your values may be different. Values may not be 100% accurate, and have not been evaluated professionally or by the US FDA.

Lunch and Dinner Recipes

Margherita Chicken

Ingredients:

1 tsp. Ground Black Pepper

1 tbsp. Fresh Basil,

1 cup Raw Spinach

4.0 oz. Chicken Breast

1/4 cup Tomato Sauce

1/4 cup Mozzarella

1/4 Garlic Clove

Directions:

1. Preheat oven to 400 degrees F.
2. Lay chicken breast between two sheets of plastic wrap and pound until 1/2 to 1/4 inch thick.
3. Season breast with pepper and salt (optional).
4. Mince garlic and sauté in olive oil for a few minutes and then add spinach and basil and sauté until wilted.
5. Lay layer of cheese on chicken breasts and then add a layer of spinach and roll each breast.
6. Put a layer of crushed tomatoes or tomato sauce on the bottom of a baking pan and sprinkle some freshly chopped basil on it.
7. Place rolled up chicken breast in the pan and then cover with the rest of the sauce on top.
8. Bake chicken breasts for 20 to 30 minutes until chicken reads a temperature of 160 F.
9. Take out the pan and place a layer of mozzarella on the breasts and sauce and broil until browned and bubbling. Temperature of chicken should reach 165 F
10. Take out and sprinkle some fresh basil on top and let cool for 5 to 10 minutes.

NOTE: Can be increased for more than 1 chicken breast.

Nutrition Facts	
Servings 1.0	
Amount Per Serving	
Calories 298	
	% Daily Value*
Total Fat 10 g	15%
Saturated Fat 5 g	23%
Monounsaturated Fat 1 g	
Polyunsaturated Fat 1 g	
Trans Fat 0 g	
Cholesterol 105 mg	35%
Sodium 941	39%
Potassium 634 mg	18%
Total Carbohydrate 12 g	4%
Fiber 4 g	14%
Sugars 5 g	
Protein 41 g	81%
Vitamin A	72%
Vitamin C	31%
Calcium	26%
Iron	19%

*Based on a 2,000 calorie diet, your values may be different. Values may not be 100% accurate, and have not been evaluated professionally or by the US FDA.

Maryland Style Broiler Crab Cakes (6 cakes)

Ingredients:

2 Large Egg

1 tsp. Worcestershire Sauce

1/2 tbsp. Old Bay Seasoning

1/4 tsp. Salt

1/4 cup Raw Celery, chopped

2 tbsp. Fresh Parsley, chopped

16 oz. Lump Crab Meat

1/3 cup Coconut Flour

1 1/2 tsp. Yellow Mustard, prepared

3 tbsp. Mayonnaise

Directions:

1. Whisk together eggs, Worcestershire, Old Bay, salt, mustard, and mayo.
2. Add celery, parsley, crab meat, and mix gently being careful not to break up crab meat.
3. Slowly incorporate coconut flour while folding the mixture.
4. Spray broiling pan with non-stick cooking spray.
5. Gently form six crab cakes and place on the pan. Refrigerate the pan for at least 30 minutes.
6. Preheat broiler and place the pan about 5 to 6 inches away from the heating element. Broil the cakes for about 8 to 10 minutes on each side, or until golden brown.

Nutrition Facts	
Servings 6.0	
Amount Per Serving	
Calories 151	
% Daily Value*	
Total Fat 8 g	12%
Saturated Fat 2 g	
Monounsaturated Fat 3 g	
Polyunsaturated Fat 3 g	
Trans Fat 0 g	
Cholesterol 125 mg	42%
Sodium 605 mg	25%
Potassium 51 mg	1%
Total Carbohydrate 4 g	1%
Fiber 2 g	10 %
Sugars 1 g	
Protein 16 g	33%
Vitamin A	4%
Vitamin C	3%
Calcium	7%
Iron	10%
*Based on a 2,000 calorie diet, your values may be different. Values may not be 100% accurate, and have not been evaluated professionally or by the US FDA.	

<u>Black and blue Burger</u>
<u>Ingredients:</u>

1/4 cup Blue Cheese

1 tsp. Ground Black Pepper

1 tsp. Ground Cayenne Pepper

1 tsp. Worcestershire Sauce

1/2 tbsp. Garlic Powder

1/4 lb. Ground Beef (95% lean)

<u>Directions:</u>

1. Light charcoal grill or gas grill and preheat. Make two zones for hot and cold grilling. (Can be pan cooked as well)
2. Mix all ingredients in a large bowl.
3. Form patty to be about ½ inch. (If making multiple burgers form more patties). Make dimple in the center of the patty.
4. Lightly oil grill grate.
5. Place burger on the hot side of the grill and cover.
6. Wait 2 minutes and flip to the other side for another 2 minutes.
7. Put burger on the cool side of the grill and cover.
8. Cook for 2-3 minutes more for medium rare burgers, 3-4 minutes for medium burgers, and 5-6 minutes more for well done.

NOTE: Serving size is one burger.

Nutrition Facts	
Servings 1.0	
Amount Per Serving	
Calories 291	
% Daily Value*	
Total Fat 15 g	24%
Saturated Fat 9 g	44%
Monounsaturated Fat 5 g	
Polyunsaturated Fat 1 g	
Trans Fat 0 g	
Cholesterol 95 mg	32%
Sodium 605 mg	25%
Potassium 598 mg	17%
Total Carbohydrate 6 g	2%
Fiber 1 g	6%
Sugars 1 g	
Protein 32 g	64%
Vitamin A	30%
Vitamin C	2%
Calcium	21%
Iron	22%
*Based on a 2,000 calorie diet, your values may be different. Values may not be 100% accurate, and have not been evaluated professionally or by the US FDA.	

Pork Quesadilla

Ingredients:

1 oz. Yellow Onion

1/2 cup Fiesta Blend

1 oz. Pickle

2 Tortillas (Low Carb Wrap)

5 oz. cooked pork (Can substitute with chicken)

Directions:

1. Spray medium sized pan with non-stick cooking spray and on medium-high heat.
2. Sauté onions and pickles until onions begin to turn translucent.
3. Add pork and heat through then turn off pan.
4. Heat a large pan on medium-high and spray with non-stick cooking spray.
5. Place one low carb wrap into the pan and heat until slightly stiff and starting to turn golden on the outside.
6. Take wrap off, re-spray pan, and put the other wrap into the pan.
7. Sprinkle half of the cheese onto the wrap in the pan, and then put the pork mixture on top of the cheese mixing lightly.
8. Sprinkle the other half of the cheese onto the pork and place the other wrap on top.
9. Flip the quesadilla and heat the other side for a moment.
10. Take off the heat.
11. Slice into pieces.

NOTE: Serving size is half of a quesadilla.

Nutrition Facts	
Servings 2.0	
Amount Per Serving	
Calories 232	
% Daily Value*	
Total Fat 11 g	17%
Saturated Fat 5 g	25%
Monounsaturated Fat 2 g	
Polyunsaturated Fat 1 g	
Trans Fat 0 g	
Cholesterol 51 mg	17%
Sodium 613 mg	26%
Potassium 73 mg	2%
Total Carbohydrate 18 g	6%
Fiber 10 g	38%
Sugars 2 g	
Protein 22 g	43%
Vitamin A	5%
Vitamin C	0%
Calcium	19%
Iron	4%

*Based on a 2,000 calorie diet, your values may be different. Values may not be 100% accurate, and have not been evaluated professionally or by the US FDA.

Broiled Pepper Jack Chicken

Ingredients:

1 tbsp. All Natural Seasoning (Roasted Garlic & Herb)

4 oz. Chicken Breast

1 Slice Pepper Jack Cheese

Directions:

1. Defrost chicken.
2. Line tray with aluminum foil and spray with cooking oil.
3. Sprinkle seasoning on to both sides of the chicken and spray the chicken with some oil.
4. Set broiler rack to about 6 inches from the heating element.
5. Turn broiler on to its highest setting and crack the oven door open.
6. Broil on each side for about 10 minutes and take it out when it reaches 160°F.
7. Pull chicken out, lay a slice of cheese on it and broil for a few minutes until it's melted.
8. Let the chicken rest for about 5 to 10 minutes.
9. Chicken should reach 165°F
10. Serve with side salad or steamed veggies

NOTE: Serving size is one chicken breast.

Nutrition Facts	
Servings 1.0	
Amount Per Serving	
Calories 169	
	% Daily value*
Total Fat 4 g	6%
Saturated Fat 1 g	6%
Monounsaturated Fat 1 g	
Polyunsaturated Fat 1 g	
Trans Fat 0 g	
Cholesterol 86 mg	29%
Sodium 1160 mg	48%
Potassium 26 mg	1%
Total Carbohydrate 6 g	2%
Fiber 0 g	0%
Sugars 0 g	
Protein 31 g	63%
Vitamin A	0%
Vitamin C	0%
Calcium	1%
Iron	4%

*Based on a 2,000 calorie diet, your values may be different. Values may not be 100% accurate, and have not been evaluated professionally or by the US FDA.

Crockpot Chili

Ingredients:

3 Green Bell Peppers

3/4 cup Beef Broth

1 tbsp. Hot Sauce

1/2 tsp. Ground Cayenne Pepper

1 tbsp. Paprika

1/4 cup Chili Powder

1 tbsp. Garlic Powder

2 tsp. Cumin Seed, whole

28 oz. Crushed Tomatoes, canned

2 lbs. Ground Beef (95% lean)

2/3 cup Onion

1 tbsp. Lime Juice, fresh

Directions:

1. Turn crockpot onto lowest setting.
2. In a large pan, brown ground beef on medium-high heat.
3. Dice bell peppers and onion into small pieces.
4. Put browned ground beef into crockpot and mix together onions and bell peppers.
5. Put remaining ingredients into the crockpot and stir together very well. Make sure to get to the very bottom and sides.
6. Cook in crock pot for at least 5 hours. Up to 8 hours is even better.
7. Serve with some sprinkled cheese on top.

NOTE: Makes about 8 1.5 cup servings

Nutrition Facts	
Servings 6.0	
Amount Per Serving	
Calories 260	
% Daily Value*	
Total Fat 8 g	13%
Saturated Fat 3 g	17%
Monounsaturated Fat 1 g	
Polyunsaturated Fat 3 g	
Trans Fat 0 g	
Cholesterol 100 mg	33%
Sodium 472 mg	20%
Potassium 785 mg	22%
Total Carbohydrate 13 g	4%
Fiber 5 g	21%
Sugars 1 g	
Protein 34 g	68%
Vitamin A	47%
Vitamin C	19%
Calcium	7%
Iron	20%

*Based on a 2,000 calorie diet, your values may be different. Values may not be 100% accurate, and have not been evaluated professionally or by the US FDA.

Smoked Sliced/Pulled Beef

Ingredients:

2 lbs. Tender Chuck Roast

2 tbsp. Ground Black Pepper

2 tbsp. Garlic Powder

2 tbsp. Worcestershire Sauce

1 tbsp. Coarse Kosher Salt

1 tbsp. Hickory Liquid Smoke

1/2 cup Beef Broth

Directions:

1. Rub salt, pepper, garlic powder, Worcestershire, and liquid smoke all over roast and place in fridge overnight to marinate.
2. Set smoker or oven to 225 F. (Hickory works well)
3. Place roast in smoker/oven uncovered and let cook until temperature reaches about 160F (about 4 to 5 hours).
4. Remove roast and place in a pan and pour beef brother over the roast and cover the pan with aluminum foil.
5. Place roast back in oven until internal temperature reaches over 200 (about another 3 to 4 hours).
6. Alternatively, this can be done in a slow cooker on low for 6-8 hours.
7. When 200 is reached, remove roast and let rest covered for 30 minutes to an hour.
8. Shred with two forks and slice any parts that don't shred easily.
9. Serve with veggies or coleslaw.

NOTE: Makes 8 (4oz) servings.

Nutrition Facts	
Servings 8.0	
Amount Per Serving	
Calories 212	
	% Daily Value*
Total Fat 13 g	20%
Saturated Fat 5 g	26%
Monounsaturated Fat 0 g	
Polyunsaturated Fat 0 g	
Trans Fat 0 g	
Cholesterol 53 mg	18%
Sodium 1785 mg	74%
Potassium 203 mg	6%
Total Carbohydrate 3 g	1%
Fiber 1 g	2%
Sugars 0 g	
Protein 20 g	40%
Vitamin A	0%
Vitamin C	0%
Calcium	1%
Iron	17%

*Based on a 2,000 calorie diet, your values may be different. Values may not be 100% accurate, and have not been evaluated professionally or by the US FDA.

Grilled Jerked Pork Chops

Ingredients:

2 tbsp. Mild Jerk Seasoning

4 Boneless Pork Chops (4oz - ½ inch)

Coarse Salt

Coarse Black Pepper

Directions:

1. Rub pork with jerk seasoning very well and let marinade overnight in the fridge.
2. Preheat grill (charcoal is best) to high heat.
3. Sprinkle salt and pepper on chops and place on hot grill to sear.
4. Cook for about 4 to 5 minutes until the chops are easily flipped and cook another 3 to 4 minutes.
5. Let rest for 5 to 10 minutes.
6. Internal temperature should reach between 145F(medium rare) and 160F(medium).
7. Serve with side salad or steamed veggies.

NOTE: Serving is one pork chop.

Nutrition Facts	
Servings 4.0	
Amount Per Serving	
Calories 291	
% Daily Value*	
Total Fat 18 g	28%
Saturated Fat 7 g	33%
Monounsaturated Fat 8 g	
Polyunsaturated Fat 1 g	
Trans Fat 0 g	
Cholesterol 93 mg	31%
Sodium 175 mg	7%
Potassium 341 mg	10%
Total Carbohydrate 1g	0%
Fiber 0 g	0%
Sugars 1 g	
Protein 30 g	60%
Vitamin A	2%
Vitamin C	5%
Calcium	0%
Iron	0%

*Based on a 2,000 calorie diet, your values may be different. Values may not be 100% accurate, and have not been evaluated professionally or by the US FDA.

Stuffed Cheesy Bell Peppers (4 peppers)

Ingredients:

4 Green Bell Pepper

1 lb. Ground Beef

1 Medium Onion

1/2 tbsp. Garlic Powder

1/2 tbsp. Ground Black Pepper

1/2 tbsp. Paprika

1/2 cup Fiesta Blend Shredded Cheese

Directions:

1. Preheat oven to 350 F.
2. Remove tops of the bell peppers and scrape out the seeds.
3. Dice the onion into small pieces.
4. In a large pan, sauté onions and brown the ground beef while seasoning with garlic powder, black pepper, and paprika.
5. Stuff each pepper with the ground beef mixture and place standing upright on a baking pan.
6. Place the pan into the oven and cook for 20 to 30 minutes until the pepper starts getting soft.
7. Remove pan and sprinkle shredded cheese on top of each pepper.
8. Put pan back in the oven for a few minutes to melt the cheese on top.
9. Remove pan and let cool for a few minutes.

Nutrition Facts	
Servings 4.0	
Amount Per Serving	
Calories 292	
% Daily Value*	
Total Fat 19 g	30%
Saturated Fat 8 g	40%
Monounsaturated Fat 8 g	
Polyunsaturated Fat 1 g	
Trans Fat 0 g	
Cholesterol 83 mg	28%
Sodium 119 mg	5%
Potassium 376 mg	11%
Total Carbohydrate 6 g	2%
Fiber 5 g	18%
Sugars 0 g	
Protein 23 g	46%
Vitamin A	10%
Vitamin C	0%
Calcium	12%
Iron	21%

*Based on a 2,000 calorie diet, your values may be different. Values may not be 100% accurate, and have not been evaluated professionally or by the US FDA.

Asian Lettuce Wraps

Ingredients:

2 cups Raw Cabbage, shredded

1/2 cup Apple Cider Vinegar (Can substitute with Rice Wine Vinegar or White Vinegar)

1/4 cup Stevia in the Raw

1 lb. Ground Pork, raw

1 tbsp. Minced Ginger

1 clove Garlic, minced

1 tsp. Mirin

1/4 tsp. Black Pepper

1 tsp. Fish Sauce

8 Whole Leaves Butter Lettuce

1/2 tsp. Salt

1/3 cup Onion

2 tbsp. Soy Sauce

2 cups Raw Carrots, strips or slices

Directions:

1. In a medium sized bowl, mix together vinegar, ¼ tsp salt, and stevia until well blended and dissolved.
2. Toss cabbage, carrots, and onion in the vinegar mixture and let sit overnight in fridge.
3. In a large pan, brown pork over medium-high heat and break up.
4. Mix in ginger and garlic and continue to cook for another 5-7 minutes.
5. Mix in soy sauce, mirin, left over salt, pepper, and fish sauce.
6. Take the pork off heat and spoon evenly into the lettuce.
7. Top each wrap with some of the carrot and cabbage mixture.
8. Fold lettuce wrap in half to eat.

NOTE: Per wrap

Nutrition Facts	
Servings 8.0	
Amount Per Serving	
Calories 209	
% Daily Value*	
Total Fat 13 g	21%
Saturated Fat 4 g	22%
Monounsaturated Fat 5 g	
Polyunsaturated Fat 1 g	
Trans Fat 0 g	
Cholesterol 53 mg	18%
Sodium 444 mg	18%
Potassium 384 mg	11%
Total Carbohydrate 9 g	3%
Fiber 1 g	6%
Sugars 3 g	
Protein 16 g	31%
Vitamin A	106%
Vitamin C	15%
Calcium	3%
Iron	6%

*Based on a 2,000 calorie diet, your values may be different. Values may not be 100% accurate, and have not been evaluated professionally or by the US FDA.

<u>**Personal Pepperoni Pizza**</u>

<u>**Ingredients:**</u>

2 tbsp. Tomato & Basil Sauce, canned

1 Pita (Low Carb)

7 slices (28g), Pepperoni

1/4 cup Mozzarella Cheese, shredded

<u>**Directions:**</u>

1. Preheat oven to 400F
2. Spread sauce evenly over pita.
3. Sprinkle mozzarella evenly over sauce.
4. Place pepperonis over mozzarella.
5. Bake on baking tray for 8-12 minutes until cheese is melted.

NOTE: For a crispier "crust" you can place the pita directly on the grate with a pan underneath.

Nutrition Facts	
Servings 1.0	
Amount Per Serving	
Calories 228	
% Daily Value*	
Total Fat 15 g	23%
Saturated Fat 7 g	33%
Monounsaturated Fat 0 g	
Polyunsaturated Fat 0 g	
Trans Fat 3 g	
Cholesterol 38 mg	13%
Sodium 848 mg	35%
Potassium 0 mg	0%
Total Carbohydrate 14 g	5%
Fiber 5 g	19%
Sugars 2 g	
Protein 16 g	32%
Vitamin A	7%
Vitamin C	7%
Calcium	21%
Iron	2%

*Based on a 2,000 calorie diet, your values may be different. Values may not be 100% accurate, and have not been evaluated professionally or by the US FDA.

Vegetable Cauliflower Fried Rice

Ingredients:

2 large Eggs

3 clove Garlic

1 cup Mixed Vegetables (Carrots & Peas)

1/4 cup Scallions

3 tbsp. Soy Sauce

2 1/2 tbsp. Sesame Oil

1 medium Cauliflower Head

Directions:

1. Chop cauliflower into smaller pieces and pulse in a food processor until the size of rice.
2. Beat eggs in small bowl.
3. Heat large wok with 1 tbsp. sesame oil over medium heat and stir fry garlic and mixed vegetables for about 5 minutes, or until vegetables are tender.
4. Mix in cauliflower, soy sauce, and the rest of the sesame oil and stir fry quickly making sure not to overcook.
5. Mix in eggs and stir in until cooked through.
6. Stir in soy sauce and green onions and serve immediately.

Nutrition Facts	
Servings 4.0	
Amount Per Serving	
Calories 174	
% Daily Value*	
Total Fat 11 g	17%
Saturated Fat 2 g	10%
Monounsaturated Fat 4 g	
Polyunsaturated Fat 4 g	
Trans Fat 0 g	
Cholesterol 93 g	31%
Sodium 792 mg	33%
Potassium 613 mg	18%
Total Carbohydrate 11 g	4%
Fiber 4 g	18%
Sugars 4 g	
Protein 9 g	17%
Vitamin A	9%
Vitamin C	137%
Calcium	6%
Iron	9%

*Based on a 2,000 calorie diet, your values may be different. Values may not be 100% accurate, and have not been evaluated professionally or by the US FDA.

Slow Cooker Buffalo Chicken Pita Wrap
Ingredients:

3 lbs. Chicken Breast

1 packet Ranch Dip Mix

12 pitas (Low Carb Pita Bread)

2 tbsp. Butter

1 (12oz) bottle Buffalo Wing Sauce

Directions:

1. Toss chicken in ranch dip mix.
2. Pour a layer of wing sauce on the bottom of slow cooker with the butter split on top of the chicken.
3. Place chicken breast into slow cooker and pour the rest of the wing sauce over the chicken.
4. Cook on lowest setting for 5-6 hours until chicken is pull apart tender.
5. Use two forks to pull chicken apart and mix well in sauce.
6. Serve on top of toasted pita with cheese, ranch, or blue cheese crumbles.

NOTE: Serving size is one wrap.

Nutrition Facts	
Servings 8.0	
Amount Per Serving one wrap	
Calories 246	
% Daily Value*	
Total Fat 7 g	11%
Saturated Fat 3 g	16%
Monounsaturated Fat 0 g	
Polyunsaturated Fat 0 g	
Trans Fat 0 g	
Cholesterol 110 mg	37%
Sodium 1919 mg	80%
Potassium 434 mg	12%
Total Carbohydrate 10g	3%
Fiber 4 g	16%
Sugars 0 g	
Protein 40 g	80%
Vitamin A	8%
Vitamin C	3%
Calcium	3%
Iron	8%

*Based on a 2,000 calorie diet, your values may be different. Values may not be 100% accurate, and have not been evaluated professionally or by the US FDA.

Baked Eggplant Parmesan

Ingredients:

3 Eggplants, peeled

2 Large Eggs

2 tbsp. Italian Seasoning

1/2 cup, Parmesan Cheese, shredded

1/2 tbsp. Ground Basil, dried

24 oz. Tomato and Basil Sauce, canned

1 1/2 cups Almond Flour

16 oz. Part-Skim Mozzarella Cheese

Salt

Directions:

1. Preheat oven to 375 F.
2. Peel and slice eggplant into ¼ inch thick slices.
3. Salt eggplant and let sit for 1 hour.
4. Pat eggplant dry.
5. Mix almond flour and Italian seasoning.
6. Beat eggs.
7. Dip eggplant slices in eggs and then in almond flour mixture coating them.
8. Bake in oven for 10 to 15 minutes flipping halfway until starting to crisp.
9. In a 9" x 13" baking dish, spread a layer of sauce on the bottom. Place layer of eggplant slices in the sauce and sprinkle with parmesan and mozzarella cheeses.
10. Repeat process again and cover top with cheeses and sprinkle dried basil on top.
11. Bake in oven for 30 to 40 minutes, or until golden brown on top.

Nutrition Facts	
Servings 12.0	
Amount Per Serving	
Calories 333	
	% Daily Value*
Total Fat 20 g	31%
Saturated Fat 8 g	42%
Monounsaturated Fat 2 g	
Polyunsaturated Fat 0 g	
Trans Fat 0 g	
Cholesterol 63 mg	21%
Sodium 853 mg	36%
Potassium 295 mg	8%
Total Carbohydrate 18 g	6%
Fiber 6 g	25%
Sugars 9 g	
Protein 23 g	46%
Vitamin A	16%
Vitamin C	8%
Calcium	55%
Iron	10%

*Based on a 2,000 calorie diet, your values may be different. Values may not be 100% accurate, and have not been evaluated professionally or by the US FDA.

Beef and Broccoli Stir Fry over Cauliflower Rice

Ingredients:

1 head Riced Cauliflower

1 1/4 cup Water

1 tsp. Xanthium Gum

3 tsp. Stevia in the Raw

1 tsp. Sesame Oil

1/2 tsp. Salt

2 tbsp. Soy Sauce

1 tbsp. Chinese Cooking Wine

1/4 tsp. Chinese 5 Spice Powder

1/4 tsp. Ground Black Pepper

4 cups Fresh Broccoli Florets

2 tbsp. Vegetable Oil (canola)

1 clove Crushed Garlic

1 tsp Fresh Ginger, grated

1 lb. Beef Sirloin

Directions:

1. In a medium sized bowl, mix together water, xanthum gum, five spice, soy sauce, stevia, sesame oil, salt, cooking wine, and pepper until thickened.
2. Slice beef into thin slices no larger than ¼ inch. (Against the grain for less chewy and with the grain for chewier).
3. Pour some sauce over beef, rub in
4. In a large wok, heat oil, sear beef quickly. May need to be done in two batches.
5. Remove beef and set aside, add ginger add broccoli to the wok, and stir fry quickly for about 30 seconds.
6. Add broccoli and stir fry quickly for about 1 to 2 minutes until tender.
7. Stir sauce and pour over vegetables and stir fry quickly until heated and starting to bubble.
8. Add beef and stir fry quickly until sauce covers everything.
9. Remove from heat and set aside.
10. Put riced cauliflower in bowl with a few drops of water, cover with paper towel,
11. Microwave 6 to 8 mins until tender.
12. Serve beef and broccoli over riced cauliflower.

Nutrition Facts	
Servings 4.0	
Amount Per Serving	
Calories 318	
	% Daily Value*
Total Fat 13 g	20%
Saturated Fat 2	9%
Monounsaturated Fat 5 g	
Polyunsaturated Fat 3 g	
Trans Fat 0 g	
Cholesterol 0 mg	0%
Sodium 832 mg	35%
Potassium 934 mg	27%
Total Carbohydrate 21 g	7%
Fiber 9 g	37%
Sugars 7 g	
Protein 31 g	62%
Vitamin A	1%
Vitamin C	55%
Calcium	165%
Iron	6%
*Based on 2,000 calorie diet, your values may be different. Values may not be 100% accurate, and have not been evaluated professionally or by US FDA.	

<u>**Chicken Fajita Wraps**</u>

<u>Ingredients:</u>

2 tbsp. Olive Oil

2 tbsp. Lemon juice, fresh

2 tbsp. Southwest Seasoning

1/2 tsp. Red Pepper Flake (optional)

1 medium Red Sweet Peppers

1 large Sweet Green Pepper

2/3 cup Onion

6 Tortillas (Low Carb)

2 lbs. Chicken Breast

<u>Directions:</u>

1. Slice chicken breast into thin strips and rub with ½ tbsp. olive oil, lemon juice, and 1 tbsp. southwest seasoning. Marinade overnight or at least a few hours.
2. Slice peppers and onion in thin strips.
3. In a large sauté pan, heat 1 tbsp. of olive oil on medium heat and sauté peppers and onions until tender and soft stirring frequently. About 10 to 15 minutes.
4. Remove peppers and onions from pan and add the last of the olive oil into the pan.
5. Turn heat up to medium-high and cook chicken until there is no pink left. About 5 to 10 minutes.
6. Once chicken is cooked, add peppers and onions back to the pan and sprinkle the remaining southwest seasoning and optional red pepper flakes and mix everything together.
7. Put tortillas in a low oven to warm up and serve by spooning the fajita mix onto the tortillas.

NOTE: One wrap is one serving.

Nutrition Facts	
Servings 6.0	
Amount Per Serving	
Calories 278	
% Daily Value*	
Total Fat 10 g	15%
Saturated Fat 2 g	11%
Monounsaturated Fat 5 g	
Polyunsaturated Fat 1 g	
Trans Fat 0 g	
Cholesterol 82 mg	27%
Sodium 489 mg	20%
Potassium 429 mg	12%
Total Carbohydrate 17 g	6%
Fiber 11 g	45%
Sugars 2 g	
Protein 33 g	65%
Vitamin A	14%
Vitamin C	84%
Calcium	5%
Iron	3%

*Based on a 2,000 calorie diet, your values may be different. Values may not be 100% accurate, and have not been evaluated professionally or by the US FDA.

<u>**Cheesy Cauliflower Crockpot Soup**</u>

<u>**Ingredients:**</u>

3 cloves Garlic

4 cups Chicken Broth

1 cup Unsweetened Almond Milk

1/2 tsp. Spices, thyme, dried

1 tsp. Salt

1 tsp. Pepper

1 1/2 cup Cheddar Cheese, diced,

2 medium Cauliflower Heads

2/3 cup Onion

<u>**Directions:**</u>

1. Dice onion and garlic into small pieces.
2. (Optional) Sautee onions and garlic on low heat until onions begin to caramelize. About 30 to 60 minutes.

Chop cauliflower roughly

3. **Place** everything but the cheese in a crockpot and cook on lowest setting until cauliflower is very tender. About 4 to 6 hours.
4. Once cauliflower is tender, use an immersion blender or regular blender and puree.
5. Once pureed, stir cheese in and serve with bacon, scallions, or anything else on top.

NOTE: Serving size is 1 ½ to 2 cups.

Nutrition Facts	
Servings 8.0	
Amount Per Serving	
Calories 168	
% Daily Value*	
Total Fat 9 g	13%
Saturated Fat 5 g	24%
Monounsaturated Fat 2 g	
Polyunsaturated Fat 0 g	
Trans Fat 0 g	
Cholesterol 31 mg	10%
Sodium 520 mg	22%
Potassium 491 mg	14%
Total Carbohydrate 10 g	3%
Fiber 4 g	14%
Sugars 4 g	
Protein 12 g	24%
Vitamin A	6%
Vitamin C	123%
Calcium	26%
Iron	5%

*Based on a 2,000 calorie diet, your values may be different. Values may not be 100% accurate, and have not been evaluated professionally or by the US FDA.

<u>**Crispy Lemon Pepper Flounder**</u>
<u>**Ingredients:**</u>

1 tbsp. Extra Virgin Olive Oil

1 Large Egg

1 tbsp. Lemon Pepper Seasoning

1 lb. (16 oz.) Flounder

1/2 cup Almond Flour

1 tsp. salt

<u>**Directions:**</u>

1. Pat flounder filets dry with paper towels and sprinkle salt over them.
2. Whisk egg.
3. Combine almond flour and lemon pepper seasoning.
4. Dip filets into egg and then coat each side with almond flour mixture.
5. Preheat olive oil in medium size pan on medium-high heat for a few minutes until the oil begins to shimmer.
6. Lay flounder filets into pan and cook each side 3 to 5 minutes until lightly golden brown.
7. Serve with lemon wedges and a side salad or steamed vegetables.

NOTE: Serving size is one filet.

Nutrition Fact 4.0s	
Servings 4.0	
Amount Per Serving	
Calories 247	
	% Daily Value*
Total Fat 18 g	27%
Saturated Fat 2 g	9%
Monounsaturated Fat 3 g	
Polyunsaturated Fat 1 g	
Trans Fat 0 g	
Cholesterol 102 mg	34%
Sodium 1178 mg	49%
Potassium 17 mg	0%
Total Carbohydrate 3g	1%
Fiber 2 g	6%
Sugars 1 g	
Protein 22 g	43%
Vitamin A	3%
Vitamin C	0%
Calcium	4%
Iron	4%

*Based on a 2,000 calorie diet, your values may be different. Values may not be 100% accurate, and have not been evaluated professionally or by the US FDA.

Garlic Herb Peppercorn Crusted Pork Loin
Ingredients:

3 lbs. Pork Loin

3 tbsp. Extra Virgin Olive Oil

2 1/2 tsp. Garlic, raw

2 tbsp. Black Peppercorn, coarse grind

2 tsp. Thyme, fresh

1 1/2 tsp. Kosher Salt

2 tsp. Sage, ground

2 tsp. Fresh Rosemary

Directions:

1. Let pork sit at room temperature for at least 1 hour.
2. Process garlic, olive oil, thyme, salt, sage, and rosemary in food processor.
3. Rub mixture all over pork loin.
4. Pat peppercorn all over pork loin.
5. Preheat broiler and place pork loin on broiling pan. Make sure the area is well ventilated or has a good vent fan in case of smoking.
6. Spray pork loin with olive oil cooking spray and set under broiling element so that it is 5 to 6 inches away from it.
7. Broil for about 10 to 15 minutes on each side until browned and internal temperature is around 145F(medium) to 160(well done). If temperature doesn't get reached and it is browning too quickly, give the loin another spray and set the rack lower. Keep an eye on the temperature when this is done.
8. Let pork rest for 5 minutes and slice. Serve with a side of vegetables or salad.

NOTE: One serving is 8 ounces or 1 cup.

Nutrition Facts	
Servings 8.0	
Amount Per Serving	
Calories 227	
	% Daily Value*
Total Fat 11 g	17%
Saturated Fat 2 g	11%
Monounsaturated Fat 4 g	
Polyunsaturated Fat 1 g	
Trans Fat 0 g	
Cholesterol 68 mg	23%
Sodium 1035 mg	43%
Potassium 7 mg	0%
Total Carbohydrate 2 g	1%
Fiber 0 g	
Sugars 2 g	
Protein 35 g	69%
Vitamin A	0%
Vitamin C	4%
Calcium	1%
Iron	7%

*Based on a 2,000 calorie diet, your values may be different. Values may not be 100% accurate, and have not been evaluated professionally or by the US FDA.